Mitral Valve Surgery

Robert S. Bonser • Domenico Pagano
Axel Haverich
(Editors)

Mitral Valve Surgery

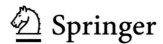 Springer

Editors
Robert S. Bonser
Queen Elizabeth Hospital
Dept. Cardiothoracic Surgeon
B15 2TH Birmingham
Edgbaston
United Kingdom
robert.bonser@uhb.nhs.uk

Domenico Pagano
Cardiothoracic Surgery
Beaumont Road 208
B30 1NX Birmingham
Bournville
United Kingdom
domenico.pagano@uhb.nhs.uk

Axel Haverich
Medizinische Hochschule
Hannover (MHH) Klinik für Herz-, Thorax-,
Transplantations- und
Gefäßchirurgie
Carl-Neuberg-Str. 1
30625 Hannover
Germany
haverich.axel@mhhannover.de

ISBN 978-1-84996-425-8   e-ISBN 978-1-84996-426-5
DOI 10.1007/978-1-84996-426-5
Springer London Dordrecht Heidelberg New York

British Library Cataloguing in Publication Data
A catalogue record for this book is available from the British Library

Library of Congress Control Number: 2010937962

Printed on acid-free paper

Springer is part of Springer Science+Business Media (www.springer.com)

Series Preface

This series is directed towards surgeons, physicians, and healthcare workers involved in the care of patients requiring cardiac, cardiothoracic, and cardiovascular surgery. The scientific developments in this field continue to be prodigious and are published in an ever-increasing journal base. We hope that the series will also provide an important resource to research workers in the quest to accelerate the translation of basic research findings into clinical study and practice. The knowledge base in our disciplines is changing rapidly and there is an important requirement to consolidate the wide-ranging information on which clinicians must base their practice.

In the series, eminent experts, serving as editors or authors, offer their accounts of innovations within our areas of practice. In some, a thorough review of the available literature is undertaken to provide a balanced reference tool for investigators to pose future research questions and understand the studies that have been previously performed to best design subsequent studies and analyses. In others, state-of-the-art, technical advances are described, affording surgeons a platform to refine their practice, providing information on thresholds of when to recommend interventions and guidance on which intervention might be appropriate.

Each and every anesthetic and surgical procedure carries a risk of mortality and complications. Much has been done to define and quantitate risk and to establish which factors may predict adverse outcome. Although such definition and quantitation may allow us to improve our counseling of patients regarding the risks of procedures, it does not necessarily allow us to categorically decide whether patients should undergo an intervention or whether they are best served by continued medical treatment or alternative modes of therapy. One of the focuses of the series will not only be the reports of which patients are at risk of which complications but will also concentrate on what avenues are available to reduce risk.

The series focuses on all aspects of cardiovascular patient care.

Some volumes will be focused on specific conditions or operative procedures while others will focus on aspects of patient care, improvements in patient management, and reduction of complications. Developments in the field are continuous and therefore, clinicians need to understand which developments in basic research can be translated into improved patient care and how these can be investigated in clinical studies and trials. This series will continue to accelerate this process, providing a detailed reference on which to base innovation and answer important clinical questions in our disciplines.

We have consciously emphasized the importance of future research direction within the series and as co-editors, we pledge to support our professional colleagues and the series readers as they share advances within our field of practice.

Birmingham, UK   Robert S. Bonser
Birmingham, UK   Domenico Pagano
Hannover, Germany   Axel Haverich

Contents

Contributors

Ottavio R. Alfieri, MD Professor and Chairman, Department of Cardiac Surgery, S. Raffaele University Hospital, Milano, Italy

Thomas A. Barker, MD, MBChB, MRCS(Ed), BSc(Hons) Clinical Lecturer in Cardiothoracic Surgery, Department of Cardiothoracic Surgery, Queen Elizabeth Hospital, Birmingham, UK

Ben Bridgewater, PhD, FRCS (CTh) Consultant Cardiac Surgeon, Department of Cardiothoracic Surgery, University Hospital of South Manchester, NHS Foundation Trust, Manchester, England

Michele De Bonis, MD Cardiac Surgeon, Department of Cardiac Surgery, San Raffaele University Hospital, Milano, Italy

Robert A. E. Dion, MD, PhD Head Department of Cardiac Surgery, Zol – Campus St. Jan, Genk, Belgium

Gilles D. Dreyfus, MD, PhD, FRCS Consultant Cardiac and Transplant Surgeon Medical Director of Cardio Thoracic Centre of Monaco, 11 bis, Avenue d'Ostende 98000, MONACO

Gébrine El Khoury, MD Professor of Cardiovascular Surgery, Pôle de Recherche Cardiovasculaire, Institut de Recherche Expérimentale et Clinique, Université catholique de Louvain, Brussels, Belgium

A. Marc Gillinov, MD Surgical Director, Atrial Fibrillation Center, Department of Thoracic and Cardiovascular Surgery, Cleveland Clinic Foundation, Cleveland, Ohio

Axel Haverich, Dr med Director, Department of Cardiothoracic, Transplantation and Vascular Surgery, Hannover Medical School, Hannover, Germany

Issam Ismail, MD, MSc Cardiac Surgery-Consultant, Division of Cardiac, Thoracic, Transplantation and Vascular Surgery, Hannover Medical School, Hannover, Germany

Chee W. Khoo, MRCP Research Fellow, University of Birmingham Centre for Cardiovascular Sciences, City Hospital, Birmingham, West Midlands, UK

Robert J. M. Klautz, MD, PhD Professor and Cardiac Surgeon,
Department of Cardiothoracic Surgery, Leiden University Medical Center,
Leiden, The Netherlands

**Gregory Y. H. Lip, MD, FRCP (London, Edinburgh, Glasgow),
DFM, FACC, FESC** Professor of Cardiovascular Medicine,
University of Birmingham Centre for Cardiovascular Sciences, City Hospital,
Birmingham, West Midlands, UK

Tomislav Mihaljevic, MD The Donna and Ken Lewis Endowed
Chair in Cardiothoracic Surgery and Staff Surgeon, Department of Thoracic
and Cardiovascular Surgery, Cleveland Clinic, Cleveland, OH, USA

Patrick Montant, MD Fellow in Cardiology, Pôle de Recherche Cardiovasculaire,
Institut de Recherche Expérimentale et Clinique,
Université catholique de Louvain, Brussels, Belgium

Agnès Pasquet, MD Associate Professor or Cardiology, Pôle de Recherche
Cardiovasculaire, Institut de Recherche Expérimentale et Clinique,
Université catholique de Louvain, Brussels, Belgium

Patrick Perier, MD Consultant Surgeon, Department of Cardiovascular Surgery,
Herz und Gefäss Klinik, Bad Neustadt/Saale, Germany

Jose Luis Pomar, MD, PhD Associate Director, The Thoracic Institute Hospital
Clinic, University of Barcelona, Barcelona, Spain

Shahzad G. Raja, MB, BS, MRCS Specialist Registrar, Department of Cardiac
Surgery, Harefield Hospital (Royal Bromptom and Harefield NHS Trust),
Harefield, Middlesex, UK

Simon G. Ray, MD Consultant Cardiologist, Department of Cardiology,
University Hospital of South Manchester, NHS Foundation Trust, Manchester, UK

Adam E. Saltman, MD, PhD Director, Atrial Fibrillation Center
and Cardiothoracic Surgery Research, Department of Cardiothoracic Surgery,
Maimonides Medical Center, Brooklyn, New York, USA

Jean-Louis Vanoverschelde, MD, PhD Professor of Cardiology, Pôle de
Recherche Cardiovasculaire, Institut de Recherche Expérimentale et Clinique,
Université catholique de Louvain, Brussels, Belgium

Francis C. Wells, MA, MS, MB, BS Consultant Cardiac Surgeon,
Department of Cardiac Surgery, Papworth Hospital, Cambridge,
Cambridgeshire, UK

Ian C. Wilson, MBCh B, MD Consultant Cardiac Surgeon,
Department of Cardiothoracic Surgery, Queen Elizabeth Hospital,
Birmingham, England

Part

I

Anatomy, Pathology, and Natural History of Mitral Valve Disease

Surgical Anatomy of the Mitral and Tricuspid Valve

1

Thomas A. Barker and Ian C. Wilson

Introduction

An appreciation of atrioventricular valve surgical anatomy reveals that they are much more than simple valves, opening and closing in response to pressure changes. The structural interrelationship of the valves of the heart and the dynamic mechanisms involved in their function are fundamental in optimizing valve performance and are dependent upon an intricate, multifaceted central cardiac complex.

The structure and physiology of this central cardiac complex combine to produce a maximal orifice area during valve opening, alongside valvular competence during ventricular systole, whilst concurrently optimizing ventricular performance. Each valve within this complex is best considered as a "Functional Unit" and any interruption of the relationships within this Functional Unit potentially results in valvular dysfunction.

The scaffolding on which the Functional Units of the atrioventricular valves are built is the fibrous skeleton of the heart; this structure stabilizes the entire central cardiac complex.

Fibrous Skeleton of the Heart

The overall structure and function of the heart depends on a widespread 'honeycomb' of connective tissue that courses throughout the heart, providing support to its cellular components.[1,2] This fine matrix is in turn supported by a more substantial network of dense connective tissue called the 'fibrous skeleton of the heart.' This fibrous structure stabilizes the base of the ventricles, thus providing a relatively inflexible, but partially deformable, scaffold for the annulus of the mitral, tricuspid, and aortic valves. The pulmonary valve is supported by the right ventricular infundibulum, and is not directly related to the fibrous skeleton of the heart.

In addition to providing mechanical support, the fibrous skeleton serves as an electrical insulator between the atrial and ventricular compartments of the heart. This electrical insulation is interrupted only at the AV node, which is situated within the center of the fibrous skeleton. A thorough comprehension of the fibrous skeleton is crucial to understanding the AV Functional Units, allowing recognition of the impact of both pathology and surgical intervention on valve function.

There are numerous components of the fibrous skeleton of the heart. The right fibrous trigone is situated at the center of the fibrous skeleton. Its superior boundary is positioned at the nadir of the noncoronary sinus of the aortic valve, whilst inferiorly it relates to the posteromedial commissure of the mitral valve. Four curved spines project from the right fibrous trigone called 'fila coronaria,' two partially surround the mitral annulus and two surround the tricuspid annulus (Fig. 1.1).

The superior, posteriorly directed limb of the fila coronaria forms the anterior mitral valve annulus and unites with the left fibrous trigone (Fig. 1.2a). The left fibrous trigone is positioned with its superior aspect at the nadir of the left-coronary sinus of the aortic valve, whilst inferiorly it relates to the anterolateral commissure of the mitral valve (Fig. 1.2b).

From the left and right fibrous trigones the fibrous skeleton extends into 'subaortic spans' creating the

I.C. Wilson (✉)
Department of Cardiothoracic Surgery, Queen Elizabeth
Hospital, Birmingham, England
e-mail: ian.c.wilson@uhb.nhs.uk

R.S. Bonser et al. (eds.), *Mitral Valve Surgery*,
DOI: 10.1007/978-1-84996-426-5_1, © Springer-Verlag London Limited 2011

Fig. 1.1 Right fibrous trigone and Fila Coronaria

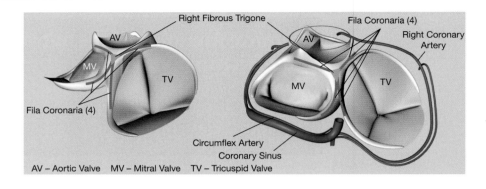

Fig. 1.2 (**a**) Superior, posteriorly directed Fila Coronaria forming the anterior mitral valve annulus and "Inter-trigonal connective tissue"; (**b**) left fibrous trigone in relation to the aortic valve

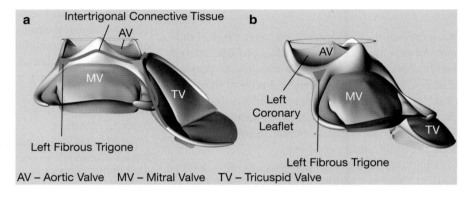

Fig. 1.3 (**a**) Aortic valve "coronet"; (**b**) "subaortic curtain"

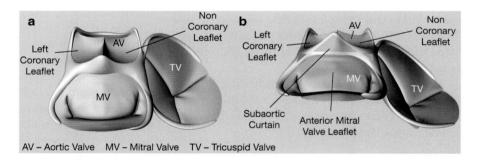

aortic annulus. These form a 'coronet' of fibroelastic tissue into which the aortic valve leaflets insert; the peak of each individual cusp within the coronet combines with the peak of the adjacent cusp to create the three commissures of the aortic valve[3] situated between the left coronary cusp, the right coronary cusp, and the noncoronary cusps, respectively (Fig. 1.3a).

The portion of the fibrous skeleton that is situated beneath the left coronary/noncoronary commissure is

referred to as the subaortic curtain, which in turn is contiguous with the fibrous skeleton of the heart. Its superior boundaries are the adjacent halves of the left coronary and noncoronary aortic valve annulus, superiorly. The curtain merges with the left and right fibrous bodies joined by inter-trigonal connective tissue inferiorly. This structure stabilizes the interaction between the two valves, referred to as the aorto-mitral continuity (Fig. 1.3b).

The anterior leaflet of the mitral valve hangs beneath the subaortic curtain, with the anterior mitral valve

Fig. 1.4 Relationship of trigones to the mitral valve commissures. (**a**) Atrial aspect; (**b**) ventricular aspect

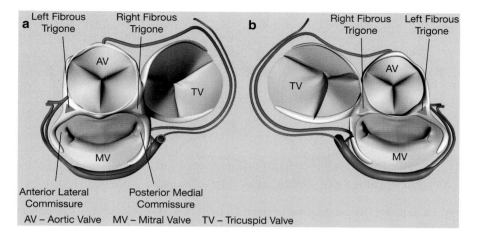

annulus formed by the inter-trigonal tissue. The right fibrous trigone supports the posteromedial commissure of the mitral valve, whilst the left fibrous trigone supports the anterolateral commissure of the mitral valve (Fig. 1.4).

The central fibrous body is the center-piece of the fibrous skeleton of the heart structurally and functionally. It consists of the right fibrous trigone, the membranous septum, and the AV node and resides at the intersection of the mitral, tricuspid, and aortic valves (Fig. 1.5). The central fibrous body serves as a central hub, providing rigid support to the entire fibrous skeleton. Age-associated calcification can occur in this area[4] which can alter its functional properties.[5] Synchronized opening and closing of these three valves is vital for coordinated cardiac function and the fibrous skeleton is fundamental in stabilizing the dynamic processes involved.

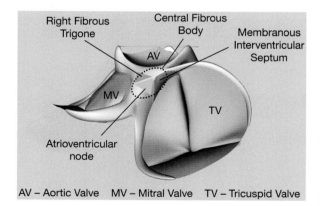

Fig. 1.5 Central fibrous body (right fibrous trigone, membranous septum, atrioventricular node)

Mitral Valve: The Functional Unit

The Structure of the Functional Unit

The mitral or left atrioventricular valve separates the left atrium and left ventricle, optimizing the antegrade passage of blood to the left ventricle during ventricular diastole, whilst preventing retrograde flow during systole. The mitral valve works as a Functional Unit, comprising numerous components, which provides the structure on which a dynamic series of physiological changes govern opening and closure throughout the cardiac cycle. The Functional Unit consists of an annulus, two leaflets, atrial myocardium, chordae tendinae, papillary muscles, and ventricular myocardium.

Surgeons and cardiologists inspect the Functional Unit of the mitral valve from different aspects. The anatomical view seen by the surgeon is visualized from the atrial aspect of the mitral valve from above (Fig. 1.6a) and has a different orientation when compared to the transesophageal echocardiographic viewpoint, which, although seen from atrial aspect of the valve, is visualized from below and is therefore simply rotated two-dimensionally by 180° (Fig. 1.6b). The transthoracic echocardiogram views of the mitral valve from the ventricular aspect is therefore a three-dimensional 180° rotation from the transesophageal echocardiogram (Fig. 1.6c). It is important to be familiar with all these views to ensure a more complete understanding of the cardiological assessment of the mitral valve, and how this relates to the anatomy encountered at the time of surgical intervention on the mitral valve.

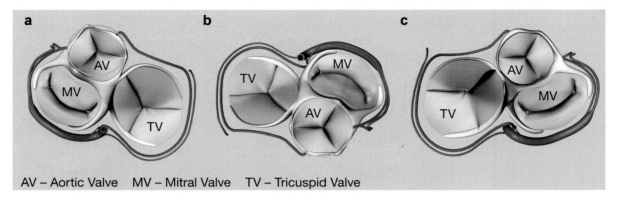

AV – Aortic Valve   MV – Mitral Valve   TV – Tricuspid Valve

Fig. 1.6 Differing views of the mitral valve. (**a**) Surgeon's view; (**b**) transesophageal transgastric view; (**c**) transthoracic parasternal short axis view

Mitral Valve Annulus

When viewed in two-dimensions the mitral annulus is asymmetrical and elliptical in shape, bearing a resemblance to a kidney bean. The anteroposterior dimension measures 0.75 of the lateral dimension. However, it has a non-planar saddle-shaped configuration, when viewed in three-dimensions, and is described as a hyperbolic paraboloid with high points anteriorly and posteriorly[6] (Fig. 1.7).

The 'fila coronaria' that surround the mitral annulus do so to a variable degree. The inter-trigonal tissue, at the base of the sub-aortic curtain is consistently present, providing a dense fibrous structure that, although not unyielding, is relatively resistant to dilatational forces. There is, however, considerable variability in the fibrous density within the inter-trigonal tissue between individuals.

The composition of the annular tissue from the left fibrous trigone, around the posterior aspect of the mitral valve annulus to the right fibrous trigone, has an even greater variability. The fibrous tissue in some mitral valves extends almost completely around the annulus with gaps filled by less dense connective tissue, whilst in others, very little fibrous extension is present beyond the inter-trigonal tissue, and trigones. In these valves the annulus is composed of areolar tissue, alongside ventricular and atrial myocardium.[7]

Annular dilatation most commonly affects the area of the mitral valve annulus least supported by connective tissue and is therefore most frequently seen within the posterior mitral valve annulus. Increases in annular

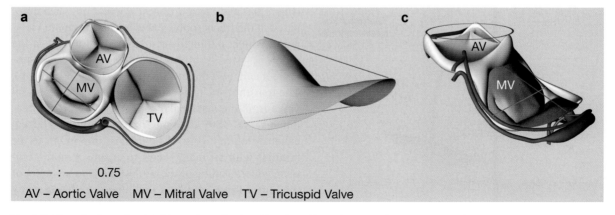

—— : —— 0.75

AV – Aortic Valve   MV – Mitral Valve   TV – Tricuspid Valve

Fig. 1.7 The mitral annulus. (**a**) Dimensions; (**b, c**) saddle-shaped hyperbolic paraboloid configuration

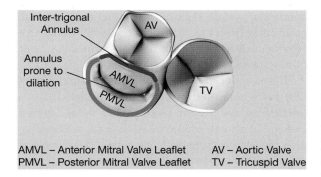

AMVL – Anterior Mitral Valve Leaflet   AV – Aortic Valve
PMVL – Posterior Mitral Valve Leaflet   TV – Tricuspid Valve

Fig. 1.8 The mitral valve annulus

dimension can lead to mitral valve insufficiency due to a consequential reduction in leaflet coaptation. It is recognized that inter-trigonal tissue dilatation can also occur, but this is both much less common and less profound (Fig. 1.8).

Mitral Valve Leaflets

The mitral valve leaflets form a continuous curtain of tissue attached to the mitral annulus that guard the left atrioventricular orifice. Although anatomical variations are reported, the mitral valve consists of two main leaflets, the anterior (aortic) and posterior (mural).

The anterior mitral valve leaflet separates the left ventricular inflow from the left ventricular outflow tract by hanging down from the fibrous skeleton between the left and right trigones. The posterior leaflet is hinged on the posterior mitral valve annulus, extending between the left and right fibrous trigones. The posterior mitral valve leaflet is attached to two-thirds of the annular circumference, whilst the anterior leaflet is attached to only a third. The junction of the anterior and posterior leaflets is formed by the mitral valve commissures. The anterolateral commissure is located beneath the left fibrous trigone, whilst the posteromedial commissure is located beneath the right fibrous trigone.

Each leaflet has three scallops, divided by sub-commissures. The posterior subcommissures are more pronounced than those on the anterior leaflet. For descriptive purposes, these scallops have been classified by Carpentier as A_1, A_2 and A_3 on the anterior leaflet, and P_1, P_2 and P_3 on the posterior leaflet. This nomenclature starts from the anterolateral commissure, A_1/P_1 and progressing across the leaflet to the posteromedial commissure, A_3/P_3.[8] (Fig. 1.9a).

The A_1 scallop, P_1 scallop and the anterolateral commissure are supported by the anterolateral papillary muscle. The A_3 scallop, P_3 scallop, and the posteromedial commissure are supported by the posteromedial papillary muscle. In contrast, the A_2 and P_2

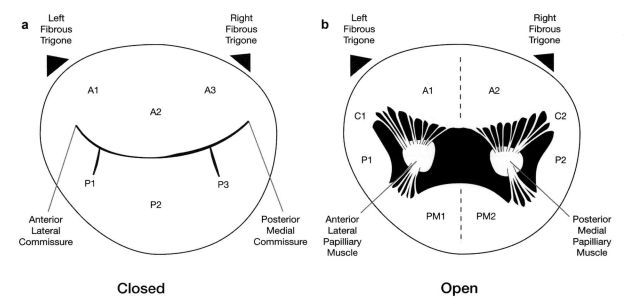

Fig. 1.9 Classification of mitral leaflet anatomy. (**a**) Carpentier's classification; (**b**) Duran's classification

scallops are supported by chordae tendinae from both papillary muscles. This distinction is important when assessing and operating on the mitral valve. This was recognized by Duran who proposed a differing classification of mitral leaflet anatomy, based on these functional considerations rather than the structural nomenclature described by Carpentier[9] (Fig. 1.9b).

The anterior leaflet is semicircular in shape with a crescentic ridge along its length. The area anterior to the ridge is called the *clear zone*, which is smooth and extends back to the annulus. Distal to the ridge is the *rough zone*, so called because of its thickened nodular surface. This nodular surface is created by the insertion points of the primary and secondary chordae tendinae. The ridge marks the "line of coaptation of the mitral valve leaflets," the site beyond which the leaflet is in contact with the posterior mitral valve leaflet when the valve is closed. The layer of coaptation between the two leaflets is known as the *zone of coaptation* (Fig. 1.10). The ratio of the rough zone:clear zone in the anterior leaflet is 0.6. The height of the anterior mitral valve leaflet ranges between 20 and 25 mm, with a width of 30–35 mm.[10–12] Although the anterior leaflet attaches to the annulus around only one third of its circumference, its surface area is larger than the posterior leaflet, and it contributes to the majority cover of the orifice area during leaflet closure.

The posterior mitral valve leaflet is hinged from two-thirds of the annulus and its three scallops P_1, P_2 and P_3 are situated opposite the corresponding three anterior divisions.[8] Although there are three scallops in 90% of cases,[13] there can be anatomical variation, with as many as five scallops reported. The middle scallop is the largest in the majority of mitral valves. The anterior mitral valve leaflet curves down to meet the posterior leaflet at the 'line of coaptation.' During

ventricular systole, the two leaflets are in contact with each other from the "line of coaptation" to the free edge of the leaflets, and this region is termed the "zone of coaptation."

The posterior leaflet is slightly different in construction when compared to the anterior leaflet. It has a rough zone and a clear zone, similar to the anterior leaflet, but also an additional basal zone, which separates the annulus from the 'clear zone'.[10,14] The ratio of rough zone:clear zone is also different when compared to the anterior leaflet (1.4), with a considerably greater proportion of rough zone within the posterior leaflet; this results from a much smaller clear zone area on the posterior leaflet (Fig. 1.11).

Mitral valve leaflets are composed of numerous layers; these are the central fibrosa and spongiosa, covered by the atrialis and ventricularis layers.

The collagenous fibrosa, together with the spongiosa, which is composed of proteoglycans, elastin, and connective tissue, makes up the core of the leaflets. The outer surfaces are composed of elastin and are named as the atrialis and ventricularis layers, with both layers covered by a layer of endothelium. Atrial and ventricular myocardium protrudes beneath the endothelial layers on the respective sides.

The fibrosa:spongiosa leaflet core demonstrates anisotropic characteristics resulting in a quasi-linear-elastic property. This results in crimping of the collagen fibers within the core of the leaflet tissue when pressure stresses are not exerted upon the leaflet. When the leaflet is exposed to stress during ventricular systole, the leaflets uncrimp, resulting in stretching out of the collagen fibers within the fibrosa and spongiosa layers, causing them to become linearly

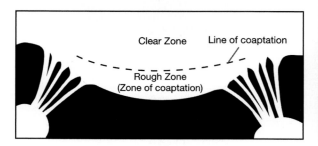

Fig. 1.10 Anterior leaflet: Rough zone and clear zone (rough: clear = 0.6)

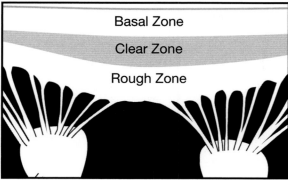

Fig. 1.11 Posterior leaflet: Clear zone, rough zone and basal zone (rough:clear = 1.4)

aligned. Subsequent pressure unloading results in recrimping. These properties of the mitral valve leaflets reduce the stresses exerted upon the leaflets during opening and closure, thereby maintaining long-term function.

Also found within the leaflets are smooth muscle cells, myocardial cells, and contractile interstitial cells. There is, in addition, leaflet neural innervation by both adrenergic and cholinergic nervous systems, both providing afferent and efferent nerves. This innervation is most prominent on the anterior leaflet on the atrial side, proximally and medially[15], and potentially plays an important role in reducing valve leaflet stress during ventricular systole by increasing leaflet stiffness, thereby maintaining long-term valve function.[16]

Mitral Valve Chordae Tendinae

The chordae tendinae connect the mitral valve leaflet to the papillary muscles. The combination of the chordae and leaflet produces a parachute-like structure during ventricular systole, which prevents regurgitation of blood into the left atrium (Fig. 1.12).

Blood passes around the chordae, after entering the left ventricle, thereby reaching the left ventricular outflow tract. The chordae arise from the apical area of the papillary muscles and most branch off either just after

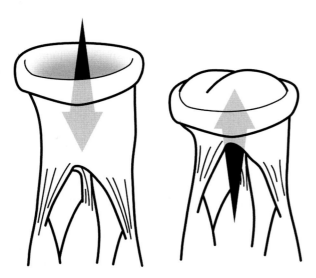

Fig. 1.12 Parachuting' of the leaflets and chordae on valve closure

their origin or just prior to insertion into the valve leaflet. They form an arcade with an origin to insertion ratio of about 5:1.[17] They are classified into 'primary,' 'secondary,' and 'tertiary' based on their points of insertion into the mitral valve leaflet.

Primary chordae, otherwise known as marginal or main chordae, insert into the free edge of the mitral valve. Commissural chordae and cleft chordae are subcategories of primary chordae. Commissural chordae insert into the free edge of the anterolateral and posteromedial commissures, whilst cleft chordae insert into the free edge of the leaflets spanning the subcommissures between the leaflet scallops. Therefore, two arrangements of cleft chordae divide the leaflets of the mitral valve into three scallops.[10]

Secondary chordae, also known as strut chordae, insert into the body of the mitral valve leaflet at the junction of the rough zone and clear zone.

Tertiary chordae originate from the ventricular muscle and insert into the base of the leaflet. Their point of insertion is into the basal zone of the leaflet and they are, therefore, not present in the anterior leaflet.

Chordae inserting into the anterolateral commissural area and the adjoining half of the two leaflets arise from the anterolateral papillary muscle. Chordae inserting into the posteromedial half of the leaflets and the posteromedial commissural area originate from the posteromedial papillary muscle. They consist of connective tissue, fibroblasts, endothelial cells, and blood vessels, exhibiting a slightly elastic property under stress. They are the narrowest, and thus the least strong, just prior to inserting into the leaflet and this is often the site of rupture.[18,19] Primary chordae are 68% thinner than basal chordae, with posterior primary chordae 35% thinner than anterior primary chordae. The anterior primary chordae are exposed to greater chordal force compared to posterior primary chordae, but these forces are considerably lesser than the forces exerted upon the respective secondary chordae.

Secondary chordae tendinae branch into three, just after they originate from the papillary muscle. They subsequently insert into the rough zone of the mitral valve leaflet. The point of insertion is into the line of coaptation, at the border of the clear zone and rough zone. These chordae are the thickest and strongest chordae. Secondary chordae are exposed to the greatest chordal force as trans-mitral pressure gradients increase during ventricular systole. The chordal force is considerably greater on the anterior secondary chordae compared to the posterior secondary chordae.

These secondary chordae play a crucial role in maintaining left ventricular geometry, and thereby preserving left ventricular contractility. Severing of the secondary chordae results in deterioration of left ventricular function, as measured by left ventricular elastance, a load-independent measure of systolic function, and preload recruitable stroke work, a load-independent measure of overall ventricular performance.

This crucial role in maintaining left ventricular geometry and function[20] underlines the importance of preserving the subvalvar apparatus when replacing the mitral valve with a prosthesis[21] and also underlines the importance of mitral valve repair, which by definition preserves the secondary chordae in almost all the cases.[22] Secondary chordal division has been proposed in surgery for ischemic mitral valve regurgitation, but this approach has not been widely embraced, in part, because of the concern about its subsequent effect on left ventricular function.

Mitral Valve Papillary Muscles

There are two major papillary muscles that stabilize the chordae tendinae during ventricular systole, which together with the chordae are known as the subvalvar apparatus. These papillary muscles are referred to as the anterolateral papillary muscle, and the posteromedial papillary muscle. The anterolateral papillary muscle is situated superiorly on the anterior wall of the left ventricle and, in 70% of cases has only one head. It is supplied by branches of the left coronary artery, either an obtuse marginal branch of the left circumflex coronary artery, or more commonly a diagonal branch of the left anterior descending coronary artery.

The posterior-medial papillary muscle is situated inferiorly on the posteroinferior wall of the left ventricle and has multiple heads, 60% of hearts having two to three heads. The postero-medial papillary muscles are supplied by branches of the right coronary artery in 85% of cases or the left circumflex coronary artery in 10–15% of cases. Acute ischemia of the papillary muscles can result in rupture leading to acute mitral valve regurgitation, whilst chronic ischemia and fibrosis can lead to papillary muscle dysfunction and chronic mitral valve regurgitation.

Physiology of the Functional Unit

Developments in magnetic resonance and ultrasound imaging have increased our understanding of the dynamic physiology within the Functional Unit. Detailed knowledge of the components contained within this intricate structure has allowed a more comprehensive insight into valvular function and dysfunction, as well as establishing the physiological consequences of surgical intervention on the mitral valve. Opening and closure of the mitral valve leaflets, within the Functional Unit, are predominantly determined by pressure changes across the valve. However, the Functional Unit facilitates valve opening and closure by alteration of annular dimensions, specific leaflet physiological properties, and subvalvar apparatus function. These factors allow optimal performance, and when not present lead to dysfunction.

Mitral Valve Annular Dynamics

The annulus undergoes significant deformation during the cardiac cycle with up to a 40% reduction in circumference during systole.[23] The annular area is largest during late-diastole, immediately prior to atrial systole, and smallest in late-systole[24] altering in size by 10–20%.[25] Left atrial systole initiates the reduction in mitral annular size prior to ventricular systole. Sixty-five percent of the reduction in annular circumference that occurs takes place prior to the onset of ventricular systole, preparing the Functional Unit for an increase in trans-mitral valve pressure gradient during ventricular systole. In a similar fashion, the increase in annular size that occurs to maximize the mitral valve area during ventricular diastole, also occurs prior to the commencement of ventricular diastole. This prepares the Functional Unit to facilitate trans-mitral blood flow; both the annular circumference and area start to increase in late ventricular systole, and are maximal just prior to atrial systole (Fig. 1.13).

In addition to changes in overall size, the annulus rotates and moves apically during systole when the ventricle shortens. This leads to a more elliptical shape thereby reducing the anteroposterior dimension of the annulus and maximizing the layer of coaptation of the mitral valve leaflets. The posterior mitral annular change is influenced by ventricular contraction.

Fig. 1.13 Annular changes during the cardiac cycle

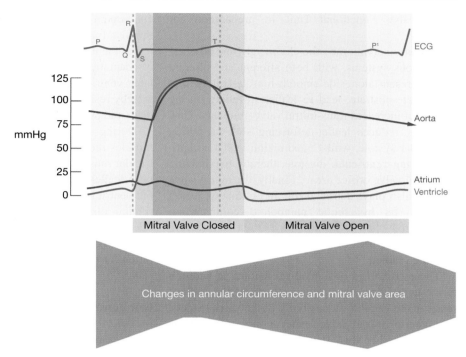

The anterior mitral valve annulus undergoes a flexible change thus buffering the differential movement between the aortic root and the posterior annulus and maintaining the left ventricular outflow tract.[26]

Mitral Valve Leaflet Physiology

Leaflet movement is also dynamic in nature, dependent on a number of physiological factors. These factors add to the ability of the Functional Unit to minimize leaflet stress and withstand increases in trans-mitral pressure gradient. The dynamic nature of these leaflet changes is influenced by many components within the mitral valve Functional Unit.

Atrial contraction plays a crucial role in preparing the leaflets for closure. Atrial contraction increases the velocity of blood flow across the mitral valve, and this increased velocity flow thereby leads to a reduction in the lateral displacement force, as determined by the principle of Bernoulli, which states that a slow-moving fluid exerts more pressure than a fast-moving fluid.

One of the most dramatic everyday examples of Bernoulli's principle can be found in the airplane, in

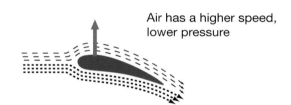

Fig. 1.14 Principle of Bernoulli

which lift occurs due to pressure differences on the surface of its wing (Fig. 1.14).

This reduction in displacement force during atrial contraction therefore allows the mitral valve leaflets to move centrally, thereby initiating the process of closure. This activity, alongside the reduction in annular size during atrial contraction, plays a huge role in optimizing mitral valve Functional Unit performance. When atrial contraction is not present, as occurs in junctional rhythm or atrial fibrillation, pre-ventricular systolic leaflet movement and annular dimension reduction, do not occur, resulting in an increased tendency to early mitral valve regurgitation.[25] The left atrial muscle, therefore, has a huge bearing on the mitral valve Functional Unit in preparation for closure.[27,28]

Leaflet innervation by the cholinergic and adrenergic nervous systems, with both afferent and efferent nerves present alongside smooth muscle cells within the leaflet substrate, lead to leaflet stiffening during periods of increased trans-mitral valve gradients. This, therefore, reduces leaflet-deforming stresses during ventricular systole, whilst maximizing leaflet compliance during ventricular diastole, thereby maximizing the mitral valve orifice area.[16] Finally, the mitral valve annulus also plays a crucial role in optimizing leaflet function. Its hyperbolic paraboloid configuration allows a reduction of the stresses exerted on the valve leaflets during periods of increased trans-mitral valve pressure gradient.[29]

These combined physiological factors, in addition to the underlying anisotropic property of the leaflets, result in the variable extensibility of the valve leaflets. The anterior mitral valve leaflet is more extensile in the radial rather than the circumferential direction, allowing increases in length of the leaflet with increased trans-mitral pressure gradients, thereby potentially increasing the zone of leaflet coaptation.

The posterior leaflet, which is hinged on two-thirds of the mitral valve annulus, is more distensible in both radial and circumferential directions, allowing both increases in posterior leaflet length, and circumference, as annular size reduces during ventricular systole. This results in greater mechanical stability of the mitral valve,[30] with an increased ability for the posterior leaflet to withstand increases in stress during periods of high trans-mitral valve gradients.

These factors are important when considering surgical intervention, and understanding the impact of disease processes on the Functional Unit. The normal layer of coaptation between the two leaflets, within the region of the rough zone, is 6–8 mm along the length of the leaflets, and is maximal between the A_2/P_2 scallops of the valve. The excess tissue found in the leaflets is almost double the area of the annulus and restoring a sufficient zone of coaptation is the primary aim of all mitral repair techniques.

Mitral Valve Papillary Muscles

Counterintuitively, papillary muscles elongate during early systole, when the left ventricular mass is contracting, and shortening. This delayed contraction, and consequent elongation, facilitates early closure of the mitral valve leaflets, ensuring early contact of the leaflets at the line of coaptation, and maximizing the zone of coaptation during early ventricular systole. During later ventricular systole, papillary muscles shorten, thereby resisting the increasing trans-mitral valve gradient and preventing leaflet prolapse.

During early ventricular diastole, the papillary muscles remain shortened, whilst the remaining ventricular muscle relaxes. This delayed relaxation facilitates leaflet opening by retracting the leaflets within the ventricle away from each other during early ventricular diastole, as the trans-mitral valve gradient opens the Functional Unit. Once the mitral valve is opened, papillary muscle relaxation occurs in preparation for the subsequent cardiac cycle.

Left Ventricular Muscle

The large posterior fascicle of the Bundle of His courses around the base of the posterior left ventricle and activates it in early systole before passing more distally. This posterior bundle activates more myocardium than the right bundle and left anterior fascicle combined and thereby provides a crucial role in coordinating the phased, activation of the ventricles. By activating the posterobasal region of the left ventricle early during this phased sequence, posterior annular changes in dimension occur early in systole. This posterior annular shortening, associated with anterior displacement, facilitates early leaflet coaptation. A loss of this early activation, as occurs with left bundle branch block, and with right ventricular pacing, potentially reduces the zone of coaptation, and increases the tendency to mitral valve regurgitation.

Summary of the Impact of Mitral Valve Physiology

Ultimately, all changes in the mitral valve Functional Unit leading up to its closure have the common aim of facilitating adequate leaflet coaptation to prevent regurgitation. The early closure of the mitral valve thereby allows isovolumetric contraction to occur, optimizing ventricular filling during this crucial phase of the cardiac cycle. Starling's Law determines that left ventricular contractility is dependent upon left ventricular filling, and mitral valve function, therefore, potentially plays a fundamental role in optimizing left ventricular contractility. This underlines the importance of ensuring early competence of the Functional Unit, and explains the complex interrelationship between the mitral valve functional Unit and overall cardiac performance.

Mitral Valve Functional Unit Co-location: Surgical Considerations

When performing mitral valve surgery, and contemplating novel percutaneous approaches to valvular repair, it is vital to have an appreciation of the structures that surround the mitral valve.

The circumflex coronary artery courses between the aorta and the pulmonary artery and continues in the left AV groove where it runs in close proximity to the posterior mitral valve annulus. In 85% of cases, its course stops here although it can extend into posterior AV groove in left dominant hearts. It gives off a variable number of obtuse marginal branches, the first of which demarcates the proximal from the distal circumflex. In the majority of cases, the left circumflex coronary artery crosses underneath the coronary sinus at a variable distance along the course of the coronary sinus.[31,32] The coronary sinus passes within the posterior AV groove, but its course is more distant to the annulus than the circumflex coronary artery. It is buried in the posterior left atrial wall above the annulus. Laterally, the coronary sinus is farthest away from the annulus, but it does course closer to the annulus posteroinferiorly (Fig. 1.15). Both of these structures are at risk of damage when operating on the posterior mitral valve annulus, particularly when complex reconstructive techniques are employed.

In addition to these vascular structures, there are other anatomical structures that are closely related to the mitral valve. The fibrous skeleton of the heart creates a layer of electrical insulation between the atria and ventricles, through which the only passage is the AV node (Fig. 1.16). The AV node is situated within the central fibrous body of the heart, with the bundles of His dividing up from this point. The small right bundle and larger left bundle exit the central fibrous body, with the left bundle dividing further into a smaller anterior fascicle and larger posterior fascicle as it passes across the membranous septum. The right fibrous trigone is an important component of the central fibrous body and is situated adjacent to the posteromedial commissure of

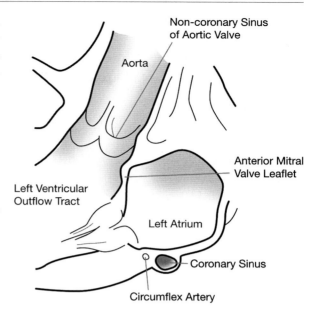

Fig. 1.15 The relationship of the coronary sinus and left circumflex artery to the mitral annulus

the mitral valve. Deep sutures within this region can result in AV node injury.

Finally, the aortic valve is in close proximity to the mitral valve. The inter-trigonal tissue within the anterior mitral valve annulus courses beneath the aortic valve leaflets, with the nadir of the left coronary sinus abutting the left fibrous trigone, whilst the nadir of the noncoronary sinus abuts the right fibrous trigone. The subaortic curtain is situated between the two trigones. The commissure between the non-coronary and left coronary cusps is, therefore, lifted away from the mitral annulus but the nadir of the left coronary cusp, and the nadir of the non-coronary cusp are in very close proximity to the mitral valve annulus. Deep sutures placed within the anterolateral and posteromedial portions of the inter-trigonal tissue can, therefore, result in injury to the aortic valve leaflets (Fig. 1.3).

Tricuspid Valve: The Functional Unit

The Structure of the Functional Unit

The tricuspid valve guards the right AV orifice, optimizing the antegrade passage of blood during ventricular diastole, whilst preventing regurgitation of blood

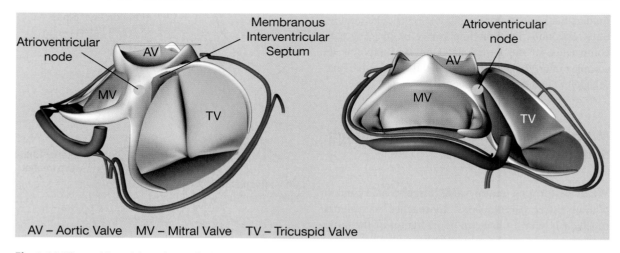

AV – Aortic Valve   MV – Mitral Valve   TV – Tricuspid Valve

Fig. 1.16 The position of the atrioventricular node

from the right ventricle to the right atrium during ventricular systole. It has many similarities to the mitral valve, although detailed knowledge of its structure and physiology is less well understood. The tricuspid valve functions as a unit with many of the same structural components as the mitral valve. This Functional Unit is stabilized by the fibrous skeleton of the heart and is seated at the level of the 'atrioventricular junction of the heart' (Fig. 1.17). Its position is anterior to the mitral valve, in a more caudal position, displaced towards the apex of the heart compared to the left AV

Functional Unit. The functional complex consists of an annulus, three leaflets, atrial myocardium, chordae tendinae, papillary muscles, and ventricular myocardium. An increasing recognition of the clinical importance of tricuspid valve dysfunction has led to an interest in understanding the workings of the right AV Functional Unit, and how they are influenced by both disease and surgical intervention.

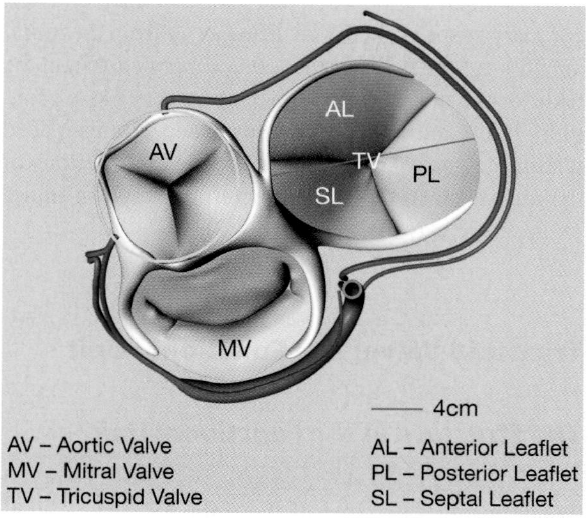

Tricuspid Valve Annulus

The annulus of the tricuspid valve is in close proximity to the central fibrous body, including both the right fibrous trigone and the membranous septum. The tricuspid annulus is oval-shaped, with its maximum end-diastolic diameter measuring up to 4cm from the septal end of the anterior leaflet to a point close to the middle of the posterior leaflet (Fig. 1.17). The annular area is about 12cm.[2,33]

The portion of the annulus adjacent to the central fibrous body is composed of fibrous tissue. This region of the annulus courses on the ventricular side of the AV junction near the membranous septum and provides a fibrous hinge for the septal leaflet on its anteroseptal half, and also fibrous attachment of anteroseptal commissure. This fibrous confluence is the core of the fibrous skeleton of the heart, at which point there is a fibrous continuity among the mitral, aortic, and tricuspid valves. However, there is septal right ventricular muscle deep to the annulus, resulting in the 'off-

AV – Aortic Valve   AL – Anterior Leaflet
MV – Mitral Valve   PL – Posterior Leaflet
TV – Tricuspid Valve   SL – Septal Leaflet

Fig. 1.17 Maximal tricuspid annular dimension

setting' of the tricuspid valve compared to the mitral valve, which lies more basally. The remaining portion of the annulus is fibroelastic areolar tissue of varying density around the annular circumference. This areolar tissue merges with both atrial and ventricular myocardium.

In a similar configuration to the mitral valve, the tricuspid valve annulus is nonplanar. The annulus is saddle-shaped with the posteroseptal and anterolateral areas being the lowest points and the posterolateral and anteroseptal portions the highest.[34,35] (Fig. 1.18).

Tricuspid Valve Leaflets

The leaflets of the tricuspid valve are thinner and less well defined than those of the mitral valve. Typically, the tricuspid valve Functional Unit has three leaflets, a septal leaflet, a posterior leaflet, and an anterior leaflet (Fig. 1.19). There is, however, considerable anatomical

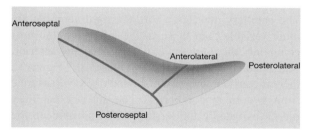

Fig. 1.18 Saddle shaped configuration of the tricuspid annulus

variation in the number of leaflets, with a range between two and six described. Leaflets are separated by commissures referred to as anteroseptal, anteroposterior, and posteroseptal.

The anterior leaflet is the largest and most mobile and is usually semicircular with a notch near the anteroseptal commissure. It extends from the anteroseptal commissure, hangs down beneath the right ventricular infundibulum, and reaches across to the anteroposterior commissure on the inferolateral wall of the right ventricle. It frequently has a large cleft functionally dividing the leaflet into two halves. In such valves, the anterior leaflet cleft is supported by subcommissural chordae tendinae (Fig. 1.20).

The anteroseptal commissure, is adjacent to the central fibrous body, and is the zone of coaptation between the anterior and posterior leaflets. The septal leaflet is attached mainly to the membranous and muscular septum, and also partially to the posterior wall of the right ventricle. It has a fold at the junction of the septal and posterior ventricular walls and also a notch near the posteroseptal commissure. This leaflet is semioval and the smallest of the three. The posterior leaflet has a variable number of clefts resulting in two to three scallops, with a range of one to four reported. The posterior leaflet runs along the posteroinferior margin of the valve.

Each leaflet is divided into three distinct zones. The 'rough zone' is between the free edge and its 'line of coaptation.' It is the chordal insertions that create the rough zone, in a similar manner to the mitral valve.

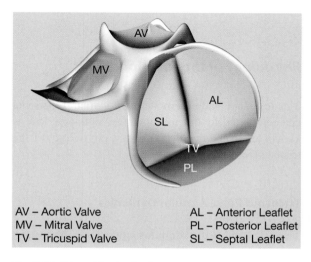

AV – Aortic Valve   AL – Anterior Leaflet
MV – Mitral Valve   PL – Posterior Leaflet
TV – Tricuspid Valve   SL – Septal Leaflet

Fig. 1.19 Tricuspid valve leaflets

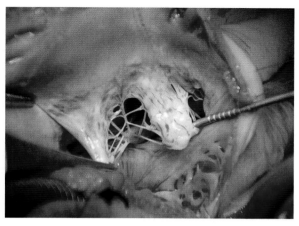

Fig. 1.20 Anatomical variation of the anterior tricuspid leaflet being divided into two halves by a cleft

The 'clear zone' passes from the 'line of coaptation' to the 'basal zone.' The 'basal zone,' which receives the basal chordae, is only a few millimeters wide. It is bordered by the 'clear zone' and the annulus.

Tricuspid Valve Chordae Tendinae

The chordae tendinae form attachments to the tricuspid valve leaflets and the right ventricular papillary muscles, acting as fibrous 'straps' which prevent prolapse of the leaflets into the right atrium during ventricular systole. The chordae of the tricuspid valve are more variable in configuration than their left-sided counterparts. Chordae tendinae originate from various points on the upper third of the papillary muscle and also directly from the anterior, posterior, and septal right ventricular wall. Chordae that branch, tend to do so shortly after leaving the papillary muscle. Primary chords remain as single chordae from source, unless they are specific cleft or commissural chords. Chordae have a similar connective tissue structure to those on the left side of the heart.

Numerous descriptions of the tricuspid chordae tendinae have been formulated. These include 'fan-shaped,' 'rough zone,' 'basal,' 'free edge,' and 'deep chordae.' However, with growing recognition of the similarities between the mitral and tricuspid valves, both functionally and when considering surgical intervention, it is logical to follow a similar terminology to that used to describe the chordae tendinae of the mitral valve. All of the previous descriptions of tricuspid valve chordae tendinae fall into the nomenclature used to define mitral chordae, although there are some differences between the chordae on two sides of the heart. Chordae tendinae are, therefore, best classified by their points of insertion into the tricuspid valve leaflet.

Primary chordae, insert into the free edge of the tricuspid valve and encompass the previously described 'free edge chordae,' as well as the specific commissural chordae, and cleft chordae, which are subcategories of the primary chordae group. Commissural, fan-shaped chordae insert into the free edge of all three commissures. Primary chordae inserting into the leaflets at sites that are not commissures or clefts are usually single, nonbranching chordae.

Secondary chordae, insert into the body of the tricuspid valve leaflet at the junction of the rough zone and clear zone. This insertion point along the 'line of coaptation' defines the clear and rough zones of the leaflets, and secondary chordae represent the 'rough zone' chordae described in previous nomenclature. In contrast to the mitral valve chordae, some 'rough zone' chordae in the tricuspid valve branch to insert into the leaflet at differing zones, including the free edge of the leaflet, the 'line of coaptation,' and the one in between these points. There is, therefore, some overlap between primary and secondary chordae within this group.

Tertiary chordae originate from the ventricular muscle, inserting into the base of the leaflet. Their point of insertion is into the basal zone of the leaflet. Tertiary chordae insert into the basal zone in half of the anterior and posterior leaflets and most septal leaflets.[36] This is in contrast to the mitral valve in which only the posterior leaflet has tertiary chordae.

Tricuspid Valve Papillary Muscles

The papillary muscles within the right ventricle are more variable than those in the left ventricle: most commonly there are three, described as the anterior, septal, and posterior papillary muscles.[37] However, there is considerable variation in number, with a range from two to nine reported. The anterior papillary muscle is usually the largest and is situated on the anterolateral right ventricular wall, whilst the septal papillary muscle is seated on the interventricular septal wall, and the posterior papillary muscle is sited posteroinferiorly.

Physiology of the Functional Unit

The tricuspid valve demonstrates similar functional characteristics to the mitral valve, although less is known about the detailed dynamic physiology of the tricuspid valve.

Tricuspid Valve Annular Dynamics

The tricuspid valve annulus undergoes significant deformation during the cardiac cycle. The tricuspid annulus is nonplanar, saddle-shaped in configuration with a more circular form during diastole, thereby maximizing the orifice area. During atrial systole, and subsequent ventricular systole, the configuration of the tricuspid valve becomes more elliptical,[38] reducing the anteroposterior dimension, thereby increasing the zone of coaptation between the larger anterior leaflet and both the septal and posterior leaflets. These changes in annular geometry result in an overall reduction of annular size by up to 40%,[39] with the annulus reaching its maximum size in isovolumetric relaxation and its minimum size in isovolumetric contraction.

The annulus normally facilitates adequate leaflet coaptation, but pathological processes can influence the relationship between the annulus and the leaflets. The portion of the annulus that abuts the central fibrous body is relatively resistant to dilatational forces, due to its fibrous composition, but the remainder of the annulus is more susceptible to dilatation as a consequence of increases in right ventricular volume. Such annular dilatation results in a reduction in the zone of coaptation of the leaflets and, when severe enough, leads to "functional" tricuspid valve regurgitation.[34,35]

Tricuspid Valve Leaflet Physiology

Tricuspid leaflet movement is influenced by the same physiological factors as the mitral valve. Early leaflet movement during atrial systole, resulting from increased blood velocity flow across the tricuspid valve, facilitates leaflet coaptation during the earliest phases of ventricular systole. This, alongside changes in annular size, due to atrial and ventricular contraction, optimizes leaflet coaptation. These factors combine to reduce leaflet stress as trans-tricuspid valve gradients increase and maintain long-term tricuspid valve Functional Unit performance.

Tricuspid Valve Papillary Muscle Physiology

Papillary muscle studies have not been performed in the same manner as they have been for the mitral valve. However, the papillary muscles have been shown to rotate with respect to the annulus during ventricular ejection.[40]

Tricuspid Valve Functional Unit Co-location: Surgical Considerations

Right Coronary Artery

The right coronary artery passes round the anterior tricuspid valve annulus in the anterior AV groove, as it courses from the right sinus of valsalva of the aortic root to the inferior aspect of the heart. The right coronary artery then gives rise to the posterior descending coronary artery in 85% of the people, which passes within the inferior interventricular groove to the apex of the heart. It is only as the posterior descending coronary artery passes into the inferior interventricular groove that the right coronary artery and its branches move away from close juxtaposition with the tricuspid valve annulus. The right coronary artery can be damaged if annular suture placement is too deep at the time of tricuspid valve surgery. The small cardiac vein also runs in the right AV groove, and can be damaged in a similar manner (Fig. 1.21).

Conduction Tissue

An integral component of the conducting system of the heart lies in close proximity to the tricuspid valve. The AV node is seated at the superior aspect of the Triangle

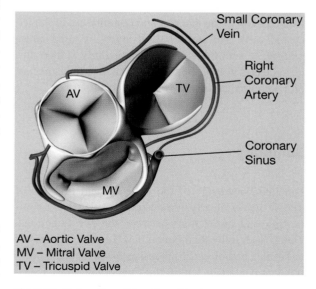

AV – Aortic Valve
MV – Mitral Valve
TV – Tricuspid Valve

Fig. 1.21 Co-location of the tricuspid valve

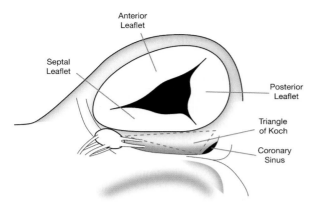

Fig. 1.22 Triangle of Koch

of Koch, is a series of superficial landmarks within the right atrium, that facilitate identification of the more deeply placed structures. The Triangle of Koch is bordered by the septal leaflet of the tricuspid valve on its left side, the coronary sinus inferiorly, and the Tendon of Todaro on its right side (Fig. 1.22). Deep to the superior apex of this triangle lays the AV node, within the central fibrous body of the heart. Deep suture placement within this region should be avoided to reduce the incidence of AV node dysfunction postoperatively.

Aortic and Mitral Valve

The noncoronary cusp of the aortic valve, and the posteromedial commissure of the mitral valve are both located deep to the anteroseptal commissure of the tricuspid valve and are at risk of injury by deep suture placement within this region, particularly if there has been destruction of the tricuspid valve annulus as part of a pathological process prior to the surgery.

Summary

Detailed knowledge of the structure and function of the AV valves clearly demonstrates considerable similarities, and interactions between the two Functional Units. Each individual Functional Unit can be exposed to similar pathological processes of the specific components contained within the Functional Unit. Trans-Functional Unit pressure gradients and ventricular

characteristics differ, but the physiological consequences resulting from cardiac disease are comparable, and are potentially treatable using similar techniques.

Similarly, the entire central cardiac complex stabilized within the fibrous skeleton of the heart can be influenced by destructive pathological processes impacting the adjacent structures, with reconstructive techniques requiring recognition of the spatial and physiological interrelationships of the Functional Units involved. A detailed three-dimensional understanding allows surgical intervention to be accomplished, preserving the relationships and thereby, the functional interdependence at the core of the heart.

References

1. Caulfield JB, Borg TK. The collagen network of the heart. *Lab Invest.* 1979;40:364-372.
2. Robinson TF, Cohen-Gould L, Factor SM. Skeletal framework of mammalian heart muscle. Arrangement of inter- and pericellular connective tissue structures. *Lab Invest.* 1983;49: 482-498.
3. Sutton JP 3rd, Ho SY, Anderson RH. The forgotten interleaflet triangles: a review of the surgical anatomy of the aortic valve. *Ann Thorac Surg.* 1995;59:419-427.
4. Tohno S, Azuma C, Tohno Y, et al. Increases of calcium, phosphorus, and magnesium in both the right and left fibrous trigones of human heart with aging. *Biol Trace Elem Res.* 2007;119:111-119.
5. Barasch E, Gottdiener JS, Marino Larsen EK, Chaves PH, Newman AB. Cardiovascular morbidity and mortality in community-dwelling elderly individuals with calcification of the fibrous skeleton of the base of the heart and aortosclerosis (The Cardiovascular Health Study). *Am J Cardiol.* 2006;97:1281-1286. Epub 2006 Mar 10.
6. Levine RA, Triulzi MO, Harrigan P, Weyman AE. The relationship of mitral annular shape to the diagnosis of mitral valve prolapse. *Circulation.* 1987;75:756-767.
7. Angelini A, Ho SY, Anderson RH, Davies MJ, Becker AE. A histological study of the atrioventricular junction in hearts with normal and prolapsed leaflets of the mitral valve. *Br Heart J.* 1988;59:712-716.
8. Carpentier A, Branchini B, Cour JC, et al. Congenital malformations of the mitral valve in children. Pathology and surgical treatment. *J Thorac Cardiovasc Surg.* 1976;72: 854-866.
9. Kumar N, Kumar M, Duran CM. A revised terminology for recording surgical findings of the mitral valve. *J Heart Valve Dis.* 1995;4:70-75. discussion 76–77.
10. Lam JH, Ranganathan N, Wigle ED, Silver MD. Morphology of the human mitral valve. I. Chordae tendineae: a new classification. *Circulation.* 1970;41:449-458.
11. Rusted IE, Scheifley CH, Edwards JE. Studies of the mitral valve. I. Anatomic features of the normal mitral valve and associated structures. *Circulation.* 1952;6:825-831.

12. Chiechi MA, Lees WM, Thompson R. Functional anatomy of the normal mitral valve. *J Thorac Surg*. 1956;32: 378-398.

13. Bezerra AJ, DiDio LJ, Prates JC. Dimensions of the left atrioventricular valve and its components in normal human hearts. *Cardioscience*. 1992;3:241-244.

14. Roberts WC, Perloff JK. Mitral valvular disease. A clinico-pathologic survey of the conditions causing the mitral valve to function abnormally. *Ann Intern Med*. 1972;77:939-975.

15. Marron K, Yacoub MH, Polak JM, et al. Innervation of human atrioventricular and arterial valves. *Circulation*. 1996;94:368-375.

16. Sonnenblick EH, Napolitano LM, Daggett WM, Cooper T. An intrinsic neuromuscular basis for mitral valve motion in the dog. *Circ Res*. 1967;21:9-15.

17. Kunzelman KS, Cochran RP, Verrier ED, Eberhart RC. Anatomic basis for mitral valve modelling. *J Heart Valve Dis*. 1994;3:491-496.

18. Sedransk KL, Grande-Allen KJ, Vesely I. Failure mechanics of mitral valve chordae tendineae. *J Heart Valve Dis*. 2002;11:644-650.

19. Lomholt M, Nielsen SL, Hansen SB, Andersen NT, Hasenkam JM. Differential tension between secondary and primary mitral chordae in an acute in-vivo porcine model. *J Heart Valve Dis*. 2002;11:337-345.

20. Goetz WA, Lim HS, Lansac E, et al. Anterior mitral basal 'stay' chords are essential for left ventricular geometry and function. *J Heart Valve Dis*. 2005;14:195-202. discussion 202–203.

21. Athanasiou T, Chow A, Rao C, et al. Preservation of the mitral valve apparatus: evidence synthesis and critical reappraisal of surgical techniques. *Eur J Cardiothorac Surg*. 2008;33:391-401. Epub 2008 Jan 14.

22. Rodriguez F, Langer F, Harrington KB, et al. Importance of mitral valve second-order chordae for left ventricular geometry, wall thickening mechanics, and global systolic function. *Circulation*. 2004;110:II115-II122.

23. van Rijk-Zwikker GL, Delemarre BJ, Huysmans HA. Mitral valve anatomy and morphology: relevance to mitral valve replacement and valve reconstruction. *J Card Surg*. 1994;9:255-261.

24. Flachskampf FA, Chandra S, Gaddipatti A, et al. Analysis of shape and motion of the mitral annulus in subjects with and without cardiomyopathy by echocardiographic 3-dimensional reconstruction. *J Am Soc Echocardiogr*. 2000;13: 277-287.

25. Timek TA, Green GR, Tibayan FA, et al. Aorto-mitral annular dynamics. *Ann Thorac Surg*. 2003;76:1944-1950.

26. Komoda T, Hetzer R, Oellinger J, et al. Mitral annular flexibility. *J Card Surg*. 1997;12:102-109.

27. Timek T, Dagum P, Lai DT, et al. The role of atrial contraction in mitral valve closure. *J Heart Valve Dis*. 2001;10: 312-319.

28. Perloff JK, Roberts WC. The mitral apparatus. Functional anatomy of mitral regurgitation. *Circulation*. 1972;46:227-239.

29. Salgo IS, Gorman JH 3rd, et al. Effect of annular shape on leaflet curvature in reducing mitral leaflet stress. *Circulation*. 2002;106:711-717.

30. May-Newman K, Yin FC. Biaxial mechanical behavior of excised porcine mitral valve leaflets. *Am J Physiol*. 1995; 269:H1319-H1327.

31. Choure AJ, Garcia MJ, Hesse B, et al. In vivo analysis of the anatomical relationship of coronary sinus to mitral annulus and left circumflex coronary artery using cardiac multidetector computed tomography: implications for percutaneous coronary sinus mitral annuloplasty. *J Am Coll Cardiol*. 2006;48:1938-1945. Epub 2006 Nov 1.

32. Tops LF, Van de Veire NR, Schuijf JD, et al. Noninvasive evaluation of coronary sinus anatomy and its relation to the mitral valve annulus: implications for percutaneous mitral annuloplasty. *Circulation*. 2007;115:1426-1432. Epub 2007 Mar 12.

33. Tei C, Shah PM, Ormiston JA. Assessment of tricuspid regurgitation by directional analysis of right atrial systolic linear reflux echoes with contrast M-mode echocardiography. *Am Heart J*. 1982;103:1025-1030.

34. Ton-Nu TT, Levine RA, Handschumacher MD, et al. Geometric determinants of functional tricuspid regurgitation: insights from 3-dimensional echocardiography. *Circulation*. 2006;114:143-149. Epub 2006 Jul 3.

35. Fukuda S, Saracino G, Matsumura Y, et al. Three-dimensional geometry of the tricuspid annulus in healthy subjects and in patients with functional tricuspid regurgitation: a real-time, 3-dimensional echocardiographic study. *Circulation*. 2006; 114:I492-I498.

36. Silver MD, Lam JH, Ranganathan N, Wigle ED. Morphology of the human tricuspid valve. *Circulation*. 1971; 43: 333-348.

37. Aktas EO, Govsa F, Kocak A, Boydak B, Yavuz IC. Variations in the papillary muscles of normal tricuspid valve and their clinical relevance in medicolegal autopsies. *Saudi Med J*. 2004;25:1176-1185.

38. Hiro ME, Jouan J, Pagel MR, et al. Sonometric study of the normal tricuspid valve annulus in sheep. *J Heart Valve Dis*. 2004;13:452-460.

39. Tsakiris AG, Mair DD, Seki S, Titus JL, Wood EH. Motion of the tricuspid valve annulus in anesthetized intact dogs. *Circ Res*. 1975;36:43-48.

40. Jouan J, Pagel MR, Hiro ME, Lim KH, Lansac E, Duran CM. Further information from a sonometric study of the normal tricuspid valve annulus in sheep: geometric changes during the cardiac cycle. *J Heart Valve Dis*. 2007;16:511-518.

Introduction

Normal mitral valve function needs structural integrity and coordinated interaction among its structures including leaflets, annulus, chordae tendinae, papillary muscles, left atrium, and the left ventricle. Mitral stenosis and mitral regurgitation are lesions used to describe cardiac dysfunction caused by structural or functional abnormalities of the mitral valve. The purposes of this chapter are to: (1) present the causes of mitral valve disease, (2) describe the structural and functional abnormalities in mitral valve disease, (3) emphasize the pathphysiologic changes in mitral valve disease, and (4) describe classifications of surgical mitral valve disease.

Mitral Stenosis

Rheumatic Mitral Stenosis

Rheumatic heart disease is the leading cause of acquired mitral stenosis. Rheumatic fever is a delayed, noninfectious consequence of pharyngitis caused by group A β(beta)-hemolytic streptococci. The World Health Organization reported an incidence of acute rheumatic fever of less than 1 case per 100,000 population per year in the industrialized world, compared to 100 to 150 cases per 100,000 population per year in some areas of eastern Mediterranean, western Pacific, and China.[1]

The rheumatic fever-induced damage is not well understood. However, evidence suggests that rheumatic fever is an autoimmune process secondary to streptococci antigen presentation. Rheumatogenic streptococci contain multiple antigenic determinants that partially mimic normal human tissue antigen.[2] In the acute phase of rheumatic valve disease, the valves are inflamed and thickened, the valve surface develops small sterile vegetations (Fig. 2.1).

The inflammatory process leads to fusion of the cusps. Valvular incompetence occurs as a consequence of thickening and distortions of the both leaflets and the chordae tendinae. In the chronic stage, rheumatic heart disease always involves the mitral valve. Aortic valve involvement is also common, but tricuspid valve involvement is less common. Mitral stenosis is caused by (1) fibrosis of the leaflets, (2) fusion of commissures, (3) fibrosis of the chordae,

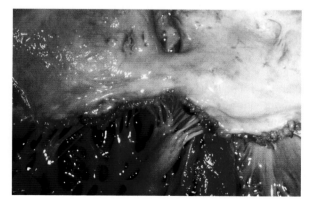

Fig. 2.1 Acute rheumatic valvulitis, mitral valve. Fibrinoid necrosis is represented by minute, translucent nodules (verrucae), 1 to 3 mm in diameter, along the lines of closure (From Wilelerson JT, Cohn JN, Wellens HJJ, Holmes DR Jr. *Cardiovascular Medicine*, 3rd ed. 2007. With permission from Springer)

I. Ismail (✉)
Division of Cardiac, Thoracic, Transplantation, and Vascular Surgery, Hannover Medical School, Hannover, Germany
e-mail: ismail.issam@mh-hannover.de

R.S. Bonser et al. (eds.), *Mitral Valve Surgery*,
DOI: 10.1007/978-1-84996-426-5_2, © Springer-Verlag London Limited 2011

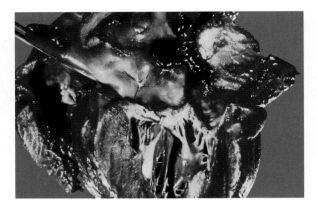

Fig. 2.2 Chronic rheumatic mitral stenosis. Note the thickening, fusion, and shortening of the chordae tendinae, as well as diffuse thickening and fibrosis of the valves, with commissural fusion. The left atrium is enlarged and contains a mural thrombus (From Wilelerson JT, Cohn JN, Wellens HJJ, Holmes DR Jr. *Cardiovascular Medicine*, 3rd ed. 2007. With permission from Springer)

and (4) subsequent calcification of the leaflets or the annulus (Fig. 2.2).

Mitral Annular Calcification

Calcification of the mitral annulus represents a degenerative disease process of the valve. Its etiology remains unclear. Mitral annular calcification is most common in elderly patients, especially in women. The calcific nodules develop in the annulus and extend to both the leaflets and to the left ventricular wall. Patients with mitral annulus calcification suffering from symptoms of mitral stenosis are at risk to develop thrombosis or infective endocarditis. Mitral stenosis in degenerative heart disease is caused by: (1) failure of annulus relaxation during diastole, (2) left ventricle LV inflow obstruction by calcific masses, and (3) narrowing of the valve orifice as a result of extension of the calcium into the leaflets.[3]

Immune Mediated Mitral Stenosis

Systemic lupus erythematosus (SLE) is an autoimmune disease affecting many organs. The etiology of SLE remains unknown, it is believed to be a result of autoantibodies to intracellular nuclear constituents,

cellular elements (red blood cells, lymphocytes, platelets, neurons or endothelial cells), and plasma components (e.g., IgG. phospholipids, clotting factors).[4,5]

The cardiac manifestations of SLE include pericardial, myocardial, and endocardial manifestations. Valvular involvement in SLE has long been recognized. Libman and Sacks, in 1924, first described a sterile verrucose endocarditis affecting the ventricular aspect of the mitral leaflets. The vegetations appear as small, flat, adherent to the valve margins, commissures of the leaflets, chordae tendinae, or papillary muscle. These lesions result in fibrous thickening and calcification of the valve and its subval-vular apparatus leading to stenosis or regurgitation (Fig. 2.3).

Rheumatoid valvular disease represents a second etiology of immune-mediated mitral stenosis and is a rare manifestation of rheumatoid arthritis. Any of the cardiac valves may be affected and various degrees of stenosis or regurgitation may ensue. Rheumatoid valvular disease is usually mild in clinical manifestation, and rarely requires surgical intervention (Fig. 2.4).

Carcinoid Heart Disease and Drug Induced Valvular Heart Disease

Carcinoid valvular disease occurs in gastrointestinal carcinoid tumors that have metastasized to the liver or to regional lymph nodes. The lesions involve particularly

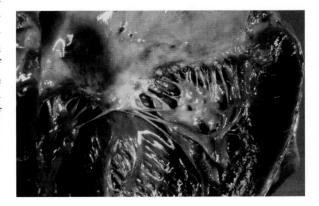

Fig. 2.3 Lupus erythematosus valvulitis (atypical verrucous endocarditis of Libman and Sacks), mitral valve (From Wilelerson JT, Cohn JN, Wellens HJJ, Holmes DR Jr. *Cardiovascular Medicine*, 3rd ed. 2007. With permission from Springer)

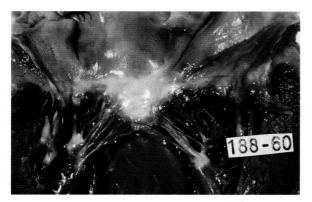

Fig. 2.4 Rheumatoid valve disease, mitral valve. Involvement may be focal or diffuse, as in this case, and is usually most prominent in the midportion of the base of the valve. The chordae tendinae are usually uninvolved, and commissural fusion is rare (From Wilelerson JT, Cohn JN, Wellens HJJ, Holmes DR Jr. *Cardiovascular Medicine*, 3rd ed. 2007. With permission from Springer)

the tricuspid and pulmonic valves. In rare cases, the left-sided valves may be affected, especially so in patients with extensive liver metastases, a patent foramen ovale, in bronchial and ovarian carcinoid.[6,7] The lesions consist of focal or diffuse, white, fibrous endocardial plaques leading to fibrosis of the valve, potentially causing stenosis or regurgitation. These lesions contain cells embedded in acollagenous stroma, which is rich in glycosaminoglycans but devoid of elastic fibers.[8,9] The secretory product responsible for development of these lesions may well be serotonin itself. The same valvular changes have been described in patients treated with methysergide and ergotamine for migraine headache, and in patients treated with the appetite suppressants, such as fenfluramine, dexfenfluramine, or the combination of fenfluramine and phentermine.

Congenital Mitral Valve Stenosis

Congenital anomalies of the mitral valve resulting in valve stenosis are rare. The supravalvular mitral ring, which is truly a circumferential ridge of endocardial thickening, is located 2–3 mm above the mitral annulus. Depending on the diameter of the ring, various degrees of obstruction may exist. More often, this ring is associated with other lesions such as a parachute or a hammock valve. It may also present as part of a complex malformation such as the Shone complex.[10]

Hypoplasia of the mitral annulus presents a rare cause of mitral valve stenosis. Commissure fusion or short chordae is another cause of congenital mitral stenosis. In this condition, one or two papillary muscles are directly connected to the commissural region of the valve without any intermediate chordae tendinae. The commissures are fused and thickened, the motion of the leaflet is restricted, and the mitral orifice is narrowed between the two papillary muscles.

Fusion of the leaflets results in two orifices or double mitral orifice. In this lesion, the interchordal spaces are obstructed by abnormal valvular tissue causing a subvalvular stenosis.[11]

The parachute mitral valve is the most common cause of congenital mitral stenosis. In this anomaly, all chordae attach to a single head or a group of posterior papillary muscles. Rarely, the entire leaflet is connected to an anterior papillary muscle. The stenosis results from obliteration of the interchordal spaces by the excess valvular tissue.[10,12,13]

Hammock valve is a term used by Carpentier to describe various subvalvular anomalies in which the central mitral orifice is partially obstructed by intermixed chordae and hypertrophied papillary muscles.[14]

Other rare causes of acquired mitral valve stenosis are amyloidosis, ochronosis, mucopolysaccharidoses, Whipple's disease, radiation, left atrial myxom or a left atrial thrombus, or active infective endocarditis with obstruction by vegetation.

Pathophysiology of Mitral Stenosis

The mechanical obstruction at the level of the mitral valve leads to obstruction of blood flow in ventricular diastole, creating a pressure gradient between the LA and the LV. The average left atrial pressure in patients with severe mitral stenosis may be in the range of 15–20 mmHg at rest, with a mean transvalvular gradient of 10–15 mmHg.[15] In addition to the severity of valvular obstruction, the transmitral pressure gradient also depends on the volume flow across the valve in ventricular diastole. For a given valve area, a higher transmitral gradient occurs with an elevated transmitral flow rate. Conversely, if cardiac output is low, only a low gradient may be present. Mitral stenosis with its resulting pathophysiology leads to morphological abnormalities of the LA, the LV, the pulmonary vascular bed, as well as the right-sided heart. Therefore, the right-side heart failure inducing tricuspid valve regurgitation often occurs as a late sequelae of chronic mitral stenosis.

The elevation of left atrial pressure leads to atrial enlargement, left atrial hypertrophy or dilatation, often in combination.[16,17] With long-standing mitral stenosis, the atrium can become massively enlarged leading to atrial fibrillation. The enlarged atrium in atrial fibrillation induces low-velocity flow patterns and atrial thrombus.

Chronic elevation of the left atrial pressure increases pulmonary vascular resistance by elevated pulmonary artery pressures. Pulmonary hypertension develops as a result of high LA pressure, pulmonary venous hypertension, and secondary pulmonary arteriolar constriction. Finally, obliterative changes in the pulmonary vascular bed with irreversible pulmonary vascular changes will occur. In mitral stenosis with subsequent LA, hypertension stands for a long time. Chronic pulmonary hypertension leads to right ventricular hypertrophy, right ventricular dilatation, tricuspid insufficiency, pulmonic insufficiency, and rightside heart failure, as often seen in cases with long-term persisting severe mitral stenosis.[18,19]

In the majority of the patients with isolated mitral stenosis and restricted left ventricular inflow, the left ventricular mass is normal or slightly subnormal.

Correction of mitral stenosis in very small LVs may result in significant postoperative dysfunction, especially in situation with postoperative volume overload.

Mitral Regurgitation

Physiological closure of the mitral valve, which prevents backflow of blood into the LA during left ventricular systole, depends on the coordinated interaction of each of the components of the valve apparatus. This consists of the LA, the annulus, the mitral valve leaflets, the chordae, the papillary muscles, and the LV.[20,21] Anatomic abnormalities or dysfunction of any one of these components may lead to valvular regurgitation. The most common disorders leading to mitral regurgitation are coronary artery disease, dilated cardiomyopathy, mitral valve prolapse, and myxomatous valve disease. Rheumatic valve disease, mitral annular calcification, infective endocarditis, congenital anomalies, connective tissue disorders, cardiac trauma, and endocardial lesions are less common causes of this pathologic entity.[22–25]

The Carpentier classification of mitral regurgitation mechanisms is based on the motion of the leaflets: Type I, normal leaflet motion; Type II, excessive leaflet motion; and Type III, restricted leaflet motion[26,27] (Fig. 2.5). Mitral regurgitation with normal leaflet motion Type I is caused by: (1) annular dilation, secondary to left ventricular dilation (patients with

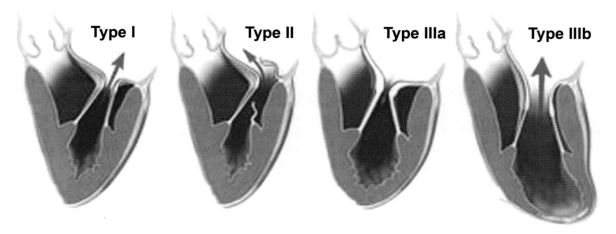

Fig. 2.5 The carpentier classification of mitral regurgitation

ischemic cardiomyopathy or dilated cardiomyopathy), or (2) leaflet perforation secondary to endocarditis.

Mitral regurgitation with excessive leaflet motion, Type II, is caused by: (1) floppy mitral valve with chordal elongation or rupture, or (2) elongation or rupture of a papillary muscle as a result of coronary artery disease. Mitral regurgitation with restricted leaflet motion, Type III, is subdivided into two types: Type IIIa based on leaflet restriction during diastole, which is seen in rheumatic disease, or Type IIIb based on leaflet restriction during systole, which is seen in ischemic mitral regurgitation.

Ischemic and Functional Mitral Regurgitation

Ischemic mitral regurgitation can be primary – organic due to a ruptured papillary muscle – or secondary – functional due to decreased myocardial function caused by ischemic heart disease. Transmural myocardial infarction can lead to partial or complete rupture of the papillary muscle or one of its heads causing acute mitral regurgitation. Papillary muscle rupture usually occurs 2–7 days after myocardial infarction. Without urgent surgery, about 50–75% of such patients may die within 24 h.[28,29] Other mechanisms include an ischemic papillary muscle that fails to tighten the chordae during systole, or a fibrotic, shortened papillary muscle fixing the chordae deeply within the ventricle.

Dilation of the LV, dilation of the annulus, apical and inferior displacement of the papillary muscles may lead to loss the coaptation of the leaflets causing functional mitral regurgitation such as in ischemic or dilated cardiomyopathy.

Functional mitral regurgitation occurs in 40% of patients with heart failure owing to dilated cardiomyopathy.[30] It is important to know that both the leaflets and the chordae are, usually, relatively normal in such cases of mitral regurgitation.

Mitral Valve Prolapse

Myxomatous degeneration of the mitral valve, also known as floppy mitral valve, Barlow disease, or mitral valve prolapse, is the most frequent cause of chronic, pure, isolated mitral regurgitation.[31] Most clinical data support the concept that mitral valve prolapse is a genetic connective tissue disorder. Recent genotypic analyses show an autosomal dominant mitral valve prolapse locus mapped to chromosome 13.[32] There appear to be at least two clinically distinct groups of patients with mitral valve prolapse.[33] The first group consists of asymptomatic younger female patients with a mid systolic click. Later, when symptoms do occur, these may be related to an associated arrhythmia or to the mitral regurgitation. The most common symptoms are palpitations, chest pain, syncope, or dyspnea. The pathologic abnormalities in this group are: (1) enlarged, thickened, opaque leaflets, (2) an increased leaflet area, (3) a dilated annular circumference, or (4) elongated and thin chordae tendinae (Fig. 2.6). Histologically, elastic fiber and collagen fragmentation as well as disorganization of these structures are present. Also, acid mucopolysaccharide material may accumulate in the leaflets.

The second group consists of older patients, typically male, with marked leaflet thickening, redundancy, and chordal rupture, associated with significant mitral regurgitation. Only 5–10% of patients with mitral valve prolapse progress to severe mitral regurgitation, and the majority remain asymptomatic. The causes of this type of severe mitral regurgitation include: annular dilation

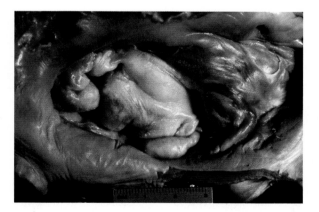

Fig. 2.6 Floppy mitral valve. The most outstanding feature is a marked increase in the surface area of the leaflets. They are voluminous, hooded, and white; however, they transilluminate with ease. Commissural fusion is not a feature of the floppy valve (From Wilelerson JT, Cohn JN, Wellens HJJ, Holmes DR Jr. *Cardiovascular Medicine*, 3rd ed. 2007. With permission from Springer)

combined with rupture or elongation of the chordae (58%), annular dilation without chordal rupture (19%), and chordal rupture without annular dilation (19%).[34]

Myxomatous degeneration of the cardiac valve, with resulting insufficiency, occurs in connective tissue disorders such as Marfan's syndrome, Ehler-Danlos syndrome, osteogenesis imperfecta, cutis laxa, and relapsing polychondritis.

Rheumatic Mitral Regurgitation

Rheumatic mitral regurgitation occurs rarely as a pure entity. In most cases, it is associated with valve stenosis and fusion of the commissures. The pathoanatomic changes in rheumatic mitral regurgitation are fibrosis of the leaflets, shortening of the chordae tendinae, fibrous infiltration of the papillary muscle, and asymmetric annular dilation. All these changes may induce loss of leaflet coaptation (Fig. 2.7).

Mitral Annular Calcification

Mitral annular calcification is most common in elderly patients. The calcification originates in the midportion of the posterior annulus, extends to the posterior

leaflets and to the left ventricular endocardium. Annular calcification usually causes mitral stenosis, but mitral regurgitation can occur by displacing and immobilizing the mitral leaflets or by impairing the presystolic sphintric action of the annulus.[3]

Infective Endocarditis

Native valve endocarditis is defined as an inflammation of the endocardium by microorganisms involving the patient's native heart valve. The most common microorganisms are streptococci and staphylococci. Gram negative bacteria and fungi also do occur, but account for only a small percentage of infective endocarditis. The hallmark of infective endocarditis is development of vegetations, usually located at the downstream side of the valve. Typically, vegetations are seen along the coaptation line of valve closure. Vegetations are variable in size but can measure up to several centimeters. Microscopically, vegetations are composed of masses of necrotic tissue, fibrin, platelets, erythrocytes, leukocytes, and infective organisms. Vegetations can cause mild mitral regurgitation by their interposition between leaflets. Severe endocarditic mitral regurgitation is usually related to a ruptured chorda, secondary destruction of leaflets, leaflet perforation, or fistula formation from a ring abscess (Fig. 2.8).

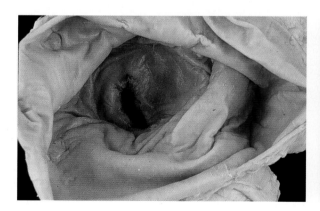

Fig. 2.7 Anatomic posterior view of the left atrium and mitral valve in a case of rheumatic mitral regurgitation. Note the wide orifice despite the presence of limited commissural fusion and note the tissue retraction leaving a wide-open orifice (From Wilelerson JT, Cohn JN, Wellens HJJ, Holmes DR Jr. *Cardiovascular Medicine*, 3rd ed. 2007. With permission from Springer)

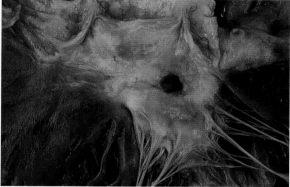

Fig. 2.8 Anatomic ventricular view of the mitral valve in a case of endocarditic mitral regurgitation with perforation of the anterior leaflet. Note the large perforation with inflammatory borders (From Wilelerson JT, Cohn JN, Wellens HJJ, Holmes DR Jr. *Cardiovascular Medicine*, 3rd ed. 2007. With permission from Springer)

Congenital Mitral Regurgitation

Congenital abnormalities of the mitral valve are not common. The atrioventricular canal defect is often associated with insufficiency of the left atrioventricular orifice. An isolated cleft of the anterior leaflet can produce important mitral insufficiency.[35] Rarer causes are double orifice mitral valve[36] and chordal agenesis.

Other rare causes of mitral regurgitation include: radiation therapy, carcinoid syndrome, methyser-gide, fenfluramine-phentermine, and endomyocardial fibrosis.

Pathophysiology of the Mitral Valve Regurgitation

Incomplete coaptation of the leaflets in the regurgitant mitral valve may create an orifice that allows passage of blood from the LV to the LA in ventricular systole. The regurgitant flow depends on the systolic pressure gradient between the LV and the atrium. This regurgitant flow is responsible for the volume overload in the LV, inducing a number of secondary morphological changes of the heart. Increased LV preload leads to changes in the left and right ventricular, as well as the left atrial, morphologies. Left ventricular pathologic changes include: (1) dilation and shape changes, (2) increased left ventricular mass, (3) hypertrophy of the LV resulting in dysfunction.[37] Chronic mitral regurgitation leads to elevated pulmonary pressure, secondary pulmonary hypertension, and right ventricular dysfunction, often in association with tricuspid regurgitation due to a dilated tricuspid annulus. These secondary changes are similar to those occurring in mitral stenosis. The LA also increases in volume. In patients, with severe, long-standing mitral regurgitation, the LA is markedly enlarged, atrial compliance is increased, and its walls may become fibrotic, but left atrial pressures remain normal or only slightly elevated for a long time.[38] The atrial fibrillation often occurs during the process of the disease.

Prosthetic Heart Valves

The most common type of valve surgery in mitral valve disease remains replacement of the diseased valve. However, mitral valve repair techniques are used at higher frequencies in recent years.

In general, restoration of a normal systolic-diastolic blood flow through the repaired or replaced valve will result not only in relief of symptoms of the patient but also in reconstructing secondary changes in the pulmonary circulation in the heart from the pathophysiological stage of mitral disease back to a normal situation. This would include relief of pulmonary hypertension, regression of left ventricular dilatation in mitral regurgitation, and increase in left ventricular volume following mitral stenosis repair. However, in cases of long-standing mitral disease and secondary pulmonary hypertension, this physiological entity may be fixed and no regression may be seen. In cases of replacement of the valve by prosthetic implants, secondary pathological changes may occur postoperatively. Mitral stenosis or incompetence is most frequently treated by excision of the diseased valve and its replacement by valve prosthesis. There are two types of heart valve prostheses: mechanical and tissue valves. Mechanical prostheses are composed of a valve body, which includes the sewing ring, a rigid, mobile occluder, and a metal cage that restricts the occluder.

Biological prostheses or tissue valves include: (1) bovine pericardial valves, (2) porcine aortic valves, (3) human dura mater or fascia lata valves, and rarely (4) homografts. The hospital mortality for mitral valve replacement with and without coronary bypass grafting has decreased. The current risk of elective primary mitral valve replacement with and without coronary bypass grafting is 5–10% in most of the studies.[39-41] The majority of deaths are due to hemorrhage, pulmonary failure, low cardiac output, and sudden death with or without documented arrhythmias. Following mitral valve replacement, the probability of 10-year survival is about 50–60%.[40-44] Autopsy studies generally reveal a higher rate of valve-related pathology than clinical investigations, 20% or more of valve recipients will ultimately die suddenly; in one autopsy study, 40% of valve recipients who died suddenly had a valve-related cause. Early prosthetic valve-associated complications are unusual. Early complications related to mitral valve insertion include dissection of the atrioventricular groove, closure of the left circumflex coronary artery by a suture, and rupture of the left ventricular free wall. Late prosthetic valve complications can be classified as follows: (1) thromboembolism and related problems, (2) infection such as prosthetic valve endocarditis, (3) structural dysfunction, and (4) nonstructural dysfunction.

Prosthetic Valve Endocarditis

Prosthetic valve endocarditis occurs in 3–6% of recipients of substitute valves and can be an early or a late complication. Early infection is defined as occurring within 60 days of valve replacement. The microbial etiology of early prosthetic valve endocarditis is dominated by the staphylococcal species (S. *epidermidis* and S. *aureus*). Late infections are related to bacteremia caused by dental procedures, urologic infections and interventions, or indwelling catheters. The most common organisms in these late infections are S. *epidermidis*, S. *aureus*, viridans streptococci, and enterococci. The infection in mechanical valves is usually localized to the sewing ring. Ring abscesses, valve dehiscence, or septic paravalvular leaks are common. Infection of the cusps may occur with tissue valves leading to cuspal perforation.

Structural Dysfunction

Structural valve degeneration is the most common cause of bioprosthetic valve failure. The probability of structural failure with currently available porcine valves remains very low in the first years after the operation but begins to increase at 8 years after surgery and reaches over 60% at 15 years.[45,46] More rapid progression is seen in children, adolescents, and dialysis patients.[45,47,48] The primary mechanism of failure is deposition of calcium phosphates in the cusp bases and in the commissures. The calcification of valve leaflets leads to stenosis, cusp perforation, and regurgitation. The incidence of structural valve degeneration is minimal for bileaflet, tilting-disk, and ball-and-cage valves.

Nonstructural Dysfunction

The most common nonstructural dysfunction is a paravalvular defect, which may be small, usually resulting from tissue contraction during healing. Large defects may follow from infection, suture knot failure, or from missing coaptation between sewing ring and native annulus in a calcified valvular annulus, as in mitral annular calcification. Severe hemolytic anemia is unusual with properly functioning contemporary valves; paravalvular leaks or dysfunction owing to

material degeneration, however, may induce hemolysis. Exuberant overgrowth of fibrous tissue, extending from the sewing ring can cause valve obstruction. This complication usually occurs late after implantation and may become clinically significant as valve obstruction, as long as 20 years after an initially successful valve implantation procedure.

References

1. World Health Organization. Rheumatic fever and rheumatic heart disease: report of a WHO Study Group. *WHO Technical Report Series*. 1988;764:1-58.
2. Stollermann GH. Rheumatogenic streptococci and autoimmunity. *Clin Immunol Immonopathol*. 1991;61:131-142.
3. Korn D, DeSanctis RW, Sell S. Massive calcification of the mitral annulus. *N Engl J Med*. 1962;267:900.
4. Arnett FC, Reveille JD. The genetics of lupus erythematosus. *Rheum Dis Clin North Am*. 1992;18:865-892.
5. Sherer Y, Gorstein A, Fritzler MJ, Schoenfeld Y. Autoantibody explosion in systemic lupus erythromatosus: more than 100 different antibodies found in SLE patients. *Semin Arthritis Rheum*. 2004;34:501-537.
6. Schweizer W, Gloor F, Von B, et al. Carcinoid heart disease with left sided lesions. *Circulation*. 1964;29:253-257.
7. Chaowalit N, Connolly HM, Schaff HV, et al. Carcinoid heart disease with primary ovarian Carcinoid ovarian tumor. *Am J Cardiol*. 2004;93:1314-1315.
8. Ferrans VJ, Roberts WC. The carcinoid endocardial plaque; an ultrastructural study. *Hum Pathol*. 1976;7:387-409.
9. Modlin IM, Shapiro MD, Kidd M. Carcinoid tumors and fibrosis: an association with no explanation. *Am J Gastroenterol*. 2004;99:2466-2478.
10. Shone JD, Sellers RD, Anderson RC, et al. The developmental complex of "parachute mitral valve" supravalvar ring of left atrium, subaortic stenosis, and coarctation of aorta. *Am J Cardiol*. 1963;11:714-725.
11. Bano-Rodrigo A, Van Praagh S, Trwitzsch E, et al. Double-orifice mitral valve: a study of 27 postmortem cases with developmental, diagnostic and surgical considerations. *Am Cardiol*. 1988;61:152-160.
12. Davachi F, Moller JH, Edward JE. Diseases of the mitral valve in infancy: an anatomic analysis of 55 cases. *Circulation*. 1971;43:565-579.
13. Moore P, Adatia I, Spevak PJ, et al. Severe congenital mitral stenosis in infant. *Circulation*. 1994;89:2099-2106.
14. Carpentier A, Branchini B, Cour JC, et al. Congenital malformations of the mitral valve in children: pathology and surgical treatment. *J Thorac Cardiovasc Surg*. 1976;72: 854-866.
15. Hygenholtz PG, Ryan TJ, Stein SW, et al. The spectrum of pure mitral stenosis. *Am J Cardiol*. 1962;10:773-784.
16. Roberts WC. Morphologic aspects of cardiac valve dysfunction. *Am Heart J*. 1992;123:1610-1632.
17. Choi BW, Bacharach SL, Barbour DJ, et al. Left ventricular systolic dysfunction: Diastolic filling characteristics and exercise cardiac reserve in mitral stenosis. *Am J Cardiol*. 1995;75:526-529.

18. Fawzy ME, Hassan W, Stefadouros M, Moursi M, Elshaer F, Chaudhary MA. Prevalence and fate of severe pulmonary hypertension in 559 consecutive patients with severe rheumatic mitral stenosis undergoing mitral balloon valvotomy. *J Heart Valve Dis.* 2004;13:942-947. discussion 947–948.

19. Schwartz R, Myerson RM, Lawrence LT, et al. Mitral stenosis, massive pulmonary hemorrhage, and emergency valve replacement. *N Engl J Med.* 1966;275:755-758.

20. Fenster MS, Feldman MD. Mitral regurgitation: an overview. *Curr Probl Cardiol.* 1995;20:193-280.

21. Hansen DE, Sarris GE, Niczyporuk MA, et al. Physiologic role of the mitral apparatus in left ventricular regional mechanics, contraction synergy, and global systolic performance. *J Thorac Cardiovasc Surg.* 1989;97:521-533.

22. Roberts WC. Morphologic aspects of cardiac valve dysfunction. *Am Heart J.* 1992;123:1610-1632.

23. Waller BF, Morrow AG, Maron BJ, et al. Etiology of clinically isolated, severe, chronic, pure, mitral regurgitation: Analysis of 97 patients over 30 years of age having mitral valve replacement. *Am Heart J.* 1982;104:276-288.

24. Waller BF, Howard J, Fess S. Pathology of mitral valve stenosis and pure mitral regurgitation, part I. *Clin Cardiol.* 1994;17:330-336.

25. Waller BF, Howard J, Fess S. Pathology of mitral valve stenosis and pure mitral regurgitation, part II. *Clin Cardiol.* 1994;17:395-402.

26. Carpentier A. Cardiac valve surgery: the French correction. *J Thorac Cardiovasc Surg.* 1983;86:323-337.

27. Carpentier A, Chauvaud S, Fabiani J, et al. Reconstructive surgery of mitral valve incompetence: ten-year appraisal. *J Thorac Cardiovasc Surg.* 1980;79:338-348.

28. Kishon Y, Oh JK, Schaff HV, et al. Mitral valve operation in postinfarction rupture of a papillary muscle: immediate results and long-term follow-up in 22 patients. *Mayo Clin Proc.* 1992;67:1023-1030.

29. Le Feuvre C, Metzger JP, Lachurie ML, et al. Treatment of severe mitral regurgitation caused by ischemic papillary muscle dysfunction: Indications for coronary angioplasty. *Am Heart J.* 1992;123:860-865.

30. Ngaage DL, Schaff HV. Mitral valve surgery in non-ischemic cardiomyopathy. *J Cardiovasc Surg.* 2004;45:477-486.

31. Hayek E, Gring CN, Griffin BP. Mitral valve prolapse. *Lancet.* 2005;365:507-518.

32. Nesta F, Leyne M, Yosefy C, et al. New locus for autosomal dominant mitral valve prolapse on chromosome 13: clinical insights from genetic studies. *Circulation.* 2005;112:2022-2030.

33. Devereux RB. Recent developments in the diagnosis and management of mitral valve prolapse. *Curr Opin Cardiol.* 1995;10:107-116.

34. Barlow JB, Pocock WA. Mitral valve prolapse, the specific billowing mitral leaflet syndrome, or an insignificant non-ejection systolic click. *Am Heart J.* 1979;97:277-285.

35. Barth CW 3rd, Dibdin JD, Roberts WC. Mitral valve cleft without cardiac septal defect causing severe mitral regurgitation but allowing long survival. *Am J Cardiol.* 1985; 55:1229-1231.

36. Rowe DW, Desai B, Bezmalinovic Z, et al. Two-dimensional echocardiography in double orifice mitral valve. *J Am Coll Cardiol.* 1984;4:429-433.

37. Zile MR, Tomita M, Ishihara K, et al. Changes in diastolic function during development and correction of chronic left ventricular volume overload produced by mitral regurgitation. *Circulation.* 1993;87:1378-1388.

38. Braunwald E, Awe WC. The syndrome of severe mitral regurgitation with normal left atrial pressure. *Circulation.* 1963;27:29-35.

39. Cohn LH, Couper GS, Kinchla NM, Collins JJ Jr. Decreased operative risk of surgical treatment of mitral regurgitation with or without coronary artery disease. *J Am Coll Cardiol.* 1990;16:1575-1578.

40. Aoyagi S, Oryoji A, Nishi Y, et al. Long-term results of valve replacement with the St Jude Medical valve. *J Thorac Cardiovasc Surg.* 1994;108:1021-1029.

41. Fiore AC, Barner HB, Swartz MT, et al. Mitral valve replacement: Randomized trial of St Jude and Medtronic Hall prostheses. *Ann Thorac Surg.* 1998;66:707-712.

42. Akins CW, Carroll DL, Buckley MJ, et al. Late results with Carpentier- Edwards porcine bioprosthesis. *Circulation.* 1990;82:IV65-74.

43. Bernal JM, Rabasa JM, Lopez R, et al. Durability of the Carpentier–Edwards porcine bioprosthesis: role of age and valve position. *Ann Thorac Surg.* 1995;60:248-252.

44. Santini F, Casali G, Viscardi F, et al. The CarboMedics prosthetic heart valve: Experience with 1084 implants. *J Heart Valve Dis.* 2002;11:121-126. discussion 27.

45. Corbineau H, Du Haut Cilly FB, Langanay T, et al. Structural durability in Carpentier Edwards standard bioprosthesis in the mitral position: a 20-year experience. *J Heart Valve Dis.* 2001;10:443-448.

46. Khan SS, Chaux A, Blanche C, et al. A 20-year experience with the Hancock porcine xenograft in the elderly. *Ann Thorac Surg.* 1998;66:35-39.

47. Borger MA, Ivanov J, Armstrong S, et al. Twenty-year results of the Hancock II bioprosthesis. *J Heart Valve Dis.* 2006;15:49-55. discussion 55.

48. Cohn LH, Collins JJ Jr, DiSesa VJ, et al. Fifteen-year experience with 1678 Hancock porcine bioprosthetic heart valve replacements. *Ann Surg.* 1989;210:435-442.

Chronic Mitral Regurgitation

3

Patrick Montant, Agnès Pasquet, Gébrine El Khoury, and Jean-Louis Vanoverschelde

Anatomy of the Mitral Valve Apparatus

The mitral valve is a complex, bi-leaflet structure that separates the left atrium (LA) and the left ventricle (LV). It consists of two leaflets, a fibrous annulus, chordae tendinae, two papillary muscles, and their left ventricular attachments (Fig. 3.1).

The annulus is composed of fibroelastic tissue, which completely encircles the valve orifice. Its general shape is that of a saddle. Seen from above, the annulus has an elliptical shape during systole and becomes more circular during diastole, reaching its maximal dimensions at end-diastole (approximately, 7.1 cm²). The annulus has two distinct functions. First, it serves as the attachment of the two mitral leaflets. Second, it exhibits sphincteric contractions during systole that decreases the size of the orifice.[1]

The two leaflets are quite different in shape. Together, they are about 2.5 times larger than the orifice, permitting large areas of coaptation. The anterior leaflet has a triangular shape and is in continuity with the aortic annulus. The anterior leaflet is juxtaposed with the non-coronary and left coronary cusps of the aortic valve. Although it encircles only one-third of the annulus, it covers more than two-thirds of the mitral orifice. The posterior mitral leaflet has a quadrangular shape. Despite the fact it occupies two-thirds of the annulus, it covers only one-third of the orifice area. The posterior mitral leaflet usually comprises three scallops, separated by clefts or indentations. In the Carpentier classification of the mitral segments,[2] the anterior or lateral scallop is usually referred to as P1, the middle scallop as P2, and the posterior or medial scallop as P3. Unlike the posterior leaflet, the anterior leaflet consists only of one large single scallop. Yet, by analogy to the posterior leaflet, it has also been segmented into three parts, mirroring the scallops of the posterior leaflet. Accordingly, the anterior or lateral part of the anterior leaflet is termed A1, its middle part is termed A2, and its posterior or medial part is termed A3. Both leaflets are thick at the bases and also at the tips, with central thinning. The anterior leaflet is more mobile, while the posterior leaflet fulfills a supporting role. The commissural areas in between the anterior and posterior leaflets are identified by the attachment of the commissural "fan" chordae. They are often referred to as Ac (anterior commissure) and Pc (posterior commissure).

The chordae tendinae are fine fibrous strings radiating from the papillary muscles and attached to corresponding halves of the anterior and posterior mitral leaflets in an organized pattern. Chordae arising from the anterior papillary muscle attach to A1 and P1 as well as to the anterior/lateral halves of A2 and P2. Chordae arising from the posterior papillary muscle attach to A3 and P3, as well as to the posterior/medial halves of A2 and P2. The chordae tendinae attach to the leaflets in three different orders.[3] First order chordae attach to the free margin of the leaflet. They are also named marginal chords. Second order chordae insert into the ventricular aspect of the leaflets. They are sometimes referred to as secondary chords. Finally, third order chordae travel from the ventricular wall and insert at the base of the posterior leaflet.

The papillary muscles are modified trabeculae that are located at the junction of the apical and middle third of the LV.[4] They always lie in a plane posterior to the intercommissural axis in diastole. The anterior papillary muscle,

J.-L. Vanoverschelde (✉)
Pôle de Recherche Cardiovasculaire, Institut de Recherche Expérimentale et Clinique, Université catholique de Louvain, Brussels, Belgium
e-mail: jean-louis.vanoverschelde@uclouvain.be

R.S. Bonser et al. (eds.), *Mitral Valve Surgery*,
DOI: 10.1007/978-1-84996-426-5_3, © Springer-Verlag London Limited 2011

Fig. 3.1 Anatomy of the mitral valve (see text for details)

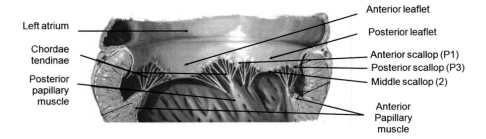

located on the antero-lateral wall of the LV usually has two well-defined heads. The posterior papillary muscle, located on the inferior/posterior wall of the LV often has three distinct heads. The anterior papillary muscle has a dual blood supply,[5] from both the first obtuse marginal branch and the first diagonal branch, whereas the posterior papillary muscle is supplied by a single artery arising from either the right coronary artery or from the third obtuse marginal of the left circumflex artery. The papillary muscles function synchronously with the LV and the chordae/leaflets to which they are attached.

Mechanisms of Chronic Mitral Regurgitation

The different elements of the mitral valve apparatus act in concert to open the valve widely during diastole and close its orifice during systole. Mitral valve closure is the result of the dynamic interaction between the annulus, which contracts early in systole, the intraventricular pressure, which acts as the closing force, the chordae tendinae, which prevent the leaflets from prolapsing into the LA, the papillary muscles, whose systolic contraction share the same purpose and the leaflets themselves, whose large apposition along the coaptation line helps reduce the stress on the leaflets and of course serves to provide continence. Disruption in any of these anatomical or physiological structures can cause mitral regurgitation (MR).

The causes of MR are numerous. From a functional point of view, they can be grouped in three main categories, as popularized by Alain Carpentier (Table 3.1).[6]

Type I dysfunction is characterized by a normal leaflet motion. In this category, MR is usually the result of annular dilation. It can also be caused by leaflet perforation or congenital anterior leaflet clefts. By itself, annular dilatation rarely causes significant degrees of

Table 3.1 Carpentier classification of mitral dysfunctions

Type I (normal leaflet motion)	Annular dilatation (LV dilatation, ischemia) (A)Leaflet perforation (endocarditis, trauma, interatrial communication ostium primum) (B) Congenital (mitral valve cleft)
Type II (increased leaflet motion)	Mitral valve prolapse (A) (Barlow (B), Marfan, Ehler-Danlos, pseudoxanthoma elasticum) Chordae rupture (C) (prolapse, endocarditis, trauma) Papillary muscle rupture (myocardial infarction, trauma) Congenital (parachute mitral valve)
Type III (decreased leaflet motion)	Leaflet retraction (A) (rheumatic fever, carcinoid tumor, systemic lupus erythematosus, systemic sclerosis, drug toxicity such as fenfluramine, phentermine, ergotamine, pergolide or cabergoline) Systolic anterior motion of the anterior leaflet (obstructive cardiomyopathy) Chordae retraction (rheumatic fever) Papillary muscle retraction and/or dysfunction (left ventricular aneurysm, myocardial infarction, ischemia, endomyocardial fibrosis) (B) Annular calcifications

MR. However, in the presence of Type II or Type III dysfunctions, progressive annular dilatation is almost always present and contributes to the progression of MR severity.

Type II dysfunction is best described as an increased leaflet motion or leaflet prolapse. There is some controversy about the definition of mitral leaflet prolapse. In the echocardiographic literature, a mitral prolapse is considered to be present whenever any part of the leaflets overrides the plane of the annulus by more than 2 mm. As the mitral annulus is saddle shaped, positive identification of a mitral leaflet prolapse requires seeing the lowest part of the annulus, which is only possible in the long-axis orientation. In the surgical literature, the definition of the mitral prolapse is more restrictive and requires part of the free edge of one (or more) of the leaflets overriding the annulus. If any other part of the valve overrides the annulus but the free edges remain above the annulus, the term billowing is then used. Type II dysfunction can be due to chordae or papillary muscle rupture, as well as chordae or papillary muscle elongation. In western countries, chordae rupture or elongation is the most frequent cause of chronic MR.

Type III dysfunction is characterized by a restrictive leaflet motion. It can be seen either when the mitral valve apparatus is affected by an inflammatory process, such as rheumatic fever (Type IIIa), or when the mitral apparatus is tethered, as in functional or ischemic MR (Type IIIb).

Pathophysiology

Determinants of Regurgitant Volume

The volume of MR depends on both the size of the regurgitant orifice and the pressure difference between the LV and the LA. Both of these two parameters vary instantaneously during systole as well as on beat-to-beat basis with the loading conditions and with LV contractility.

Instantaneous systolic variations in the regurgitant orifice mainly depend on the type of mitral dysfunction (Table 3.1).[7] In Type II dysfunction, both the instantaneous MR orifice and MR volume are maximal in late systole, when the mitral valve prolapse is the greatest. In Type IIIa dysfunction, like in rheumatic MR, the MR orifice is usually fixed so that the instantaneous changes in MR flow rate and volume are strictly LV pressure dependent. Finally, in ischemic or functional MR (Type IIIb dysfunction), the regurgitant orifice is usually the largest in early and late systole and can be almost virtual in mid-systole.

Increases in both preload and afterload and depression of contractility increase LV size and enlarge the mitral annulus on a beat-to-beat basis and increase thereby the regurgitant orifice. By contrast, increases in contractility, brought about for instance by positive inotropic agents, decreases in preload, for instance as a result of diuretics, and decreases in afterload, as seen with vasodilators, reduce the size of the LV and of the mitral annulus leading to a decrease in the size of both the regurgitant orifice and the RV.

LV Mechanics in MR

Because MR starts as soon as the LV pressure rises, almost 50% of the RV is ejected into the LA before the aortic valve opens. Once the aortic valve is opened, the LV continues to empty in both the aorta and the LA. As the impedance to ejection is considerably smaller towards the LA (because the regurgitant mitral orifice lies in parallel to the aortic orifice and because LA pressure is five- to tenfold lower than aortic pressure), the impedance to LV ejection and, hence, afterload is reduced in patients with MR. This permits maintenance of LV ejection fraction (LVEF) in the normal to supranormal range.[8] The reduced LV afterload also allows for a greater proportion of the myocardial contractile energy to be expended in shortening than in tension development, which explains why myocardial oxygen consumption and coronary flow rates are seldom increased in patients with severe MR.

LV Compensation

To maintain resting forward stroke volume, the LV compensates for the development of MR both by emptying more completely and by increasing its end-diastolic volume. By means of the Laplace law, the larger ventricular end-diastolic volume increases diastolic wall tension. In the early stages of the disease process, this triggers the release of mast cell secretagogues, such as endothelin-1, that cause mast cell degranulation.[9] In turn, mast cell secretory products, such as tryptase, chymase or TNF-α stimulate immature resident mast cell maturation and cause the activation of the matrix metalloproteinases (MMP). The resulting degradation of extracellular matrix proteins (ECM) produces side-to-side slippage of cardiac myocytes, the hallmark of ventricular remodeling. In this process, the predominant Type I collagen fibers are progressively replaced by more compliant Type III collagen fibers, which possess less cross-linking. This contributes to the reduction in LV diastolic stiffness and to the characteristic shift to the right (greater volume at any pressure) in the LV diastolic pressure-volume curve.[9]

In addition to these structural changes, there is development of a typical volume overload (eccentric) hypertrophy, in which myocytes elongate and new sarcomeres are laid down in series.[10] The eccentric hypertrophy seen in MR has been shown to be improved by β-adrenergic receptor blockade but not by angiotensin-converting enzyme inhibition or angiotensin Type I receptor blockade, suggesting that the adrenergic system is more central to the pathophysiology of the volume overload hypertrophy seen in MR.[11] It is noteworthy that the degree of hypertrophy is often not proportionate to the degree of LV dilation, so that the ratio of LV mass to end-diastolic volume may be less than normal.

In most patients, LA pressure remains normal or is only slightly elevated. Long-standing MR in these patients has altered the physical properties of the LA wall and has displaced the atrial pressure–volume curve to the right, allowing for a normal or almost normal pressure to exist in a greatly enlarged LA.

LV Decompensation

In the compensated phase of volume overload, the stressed ventricle initially exhibits adequate function, normal shape, and a normal or slightly reduced ventricular mass-to-volume ratio. At some point in time, the compensatory ability of the heart is exhausted and the heart begins to fail. At this stage, ventricular wall thickness is disproportionately reduced relative to an increased chamber volume, and ventricular shape tends to become spherical. End-systolic volume, preload, and afterload all rise, ejection fraction and stroke volume decline and chamber stiffness increases. In such patients, there is evidence of neurohormonal activation and elevation of circulating proinflammatory cytokines. Plasma brain natriuretic peptide (BNP) levels also increase, albeit to a larger extent in patients with symptomatic decompensation.[12]

Although the exact mechanisms underlying the transition from compensated to decompensated volume overload hypertrophy are poorly understood, it seems that progressive increases in MR volume play an important role. Indeed, MR is a dynamic process that constantly aggravates with time.[13] The increase in LV end-diastolic volume that accompanies significant MR causes the mitral annulus to increase in size, which in turn aggravates the severity of MR and creates a vicious circle in which "MR begets more MR."

Epidemiology

The prevalence of MR varies inversely with its severity.[14–16] A trivial MR is detectable by color Doppler echocardiography in up to 70% of normal adults. In the Framingham Heart Study, MR of at least mild severity was present on color Doppler echocardiography in 19% of the population.[15] Finally, in the Strong Heart Study, moderate or severe MR was found in 1.9% and 0.2%, respectively.[15] The estimated prevalence of mitral valve prolapse (MVP) using echocardiography is 0.6–2.4 %.[17,18]

Symptoms

Most patients with severe MR long remain asymptomatic. When present, the severity of the symptoms is related to the severity of regurgitation, its rate of progression, the pulmonary artery pressure, and to associated cardiac diseases and complications of MR.

Exertional dyspnea and fatigue, secondary to the decreased forward cardiac output and the increased LA pressure, are the commonest symptoms. The presence of symptoms plays a major role in the decision between medical and surgical management. In other words, truly asymptomatic patients must be differentiated from patients who have adapted their daily activities not to feel symptomatic. Another common symptom is intermittent or persistent atrial fibrillation(AF).

Patients with more advanced and severe disease eventually progress to symptomatic heart failure with pulmonary congestion and peripheral edema. Finally, symptoms may be related to complications of MR such as thromboembolism due to AF, hemoptysis, right-sided heart failure, and endocarditis.

Physical Examination

The systolic murmur is the most prominent physical finding in patients with severe MR. In most patients, the murmur starts immediately after a soft S1 and continues beyond A2 because of the persisting pressure difference between the LV and the LA after aortic valve closure. The murmur of chronic MR is usually constant in intensity, blowing, high-pitched, and loudest at the apex with frequent radiation to the left axilla. However, radiation toward the aortic area may occur when MR is caused by a posterior leaflet prolapse. The murmur shows little change in intensity even in the presence of large beat-to-beat variations of LV stroke volume, such as those that occur in AF. There is also a little correlation between the intensity of the murmur and the severity of MR.[19]

The MR murmur may be holosystolic, late systolic, or early systolic. When the murmur is confined to late systole, as occurs in patients with mitral valve prolapse or papillary muscle dysfunction, the regurgitation is usually not severe. These causes of MR are frequently associated with a normal S1 because initial closure of the mitral leaflets is unimpaired. A midsystolic click preceding a mid-to-late systolic murmur, helps to establish the diagnosis of mitral valve prolapse.

When chronic severe MR is caused by defective valve leaflets, S1, produced by mitral valve closure, is usually diminished. Wide splitting of S2 is common and results from the shortening of LV ejection and an earlier A2 as a consequence of reduced resistance to LV ejection. In patients with severe pulmonary hypertension (PHT), P2 is louder than A2. The abnormal increase in the flow rate across the mitral orifice during the rapid filling phase is often associated with an S3.

Laboratory Investigations

Electrocardiography

The electrocardiographic features associated with chronic MR are LA enlargement (P wave > 120 ms in lead II with a negative component in V1 > 40 ms), AF, and LV hypertrophy (increased QRS amplitude, ST-T wave abnormalities). Later, once PHT occurs, there may be evidence of right ventricular hypertrophy (tall R wave in V1 or V2 with R/S ratio >1).

Chest Roentgenogram

Cardiomegaly is the most common finding on the chest roentgenogram, resulting from both LV and LA enlargement. Signs of heart failure may be present (Kerley B lines, peribronchial cuffing, enlargement of the pulmonary vessels in the upper lung zones, hilar enlargement, and pleural effusion). In older patients as well as in Barlow's disease, a calcified mitral annulus can be seen.

Echocardiography

Echocardiography is essential for establishing the presence of MR, quantitating its severity and hemodynamic consequences, determining its etiology, and assessing the potential for repairability.[20,21]

The severity of MR should be evaluated using an integrated approach that includes valve morphology, the size of the regurgitant jet in the LA, the proximal regurgitant jet width or vena contracta, the pulmonary venous flow pattern and the measurement of the effective regurgitant orifice area (EROA), and the RV.[22]

The *Color jet area* is more useful in evaluating the mechanisms of MR than in quantifying its severity. Although semiquantification of MR severity is feasible using this approach, it is often poorly accurate, as the extension of the jet into the LA is equally impacted by physiological factors, such as blood pressure, and instrument settings, such as gain, transmit power and pulse repetition frequency, as by MR severity itself.

The *pulmonary vein flow pattern* can provide information on the hemodynamic impact of MR but is purely qualitative and is affected by many factors (AF, LV dysfunction).

Measurement of the *vena contracta* width provides quantitative data on the size of the regurgitant orifice and, hence, on the severity of MR. The vena contracta corresponds to the narrowest segment of the jet on color flow imaging. Values exceeding 7 mm are usually associated with severe MR.

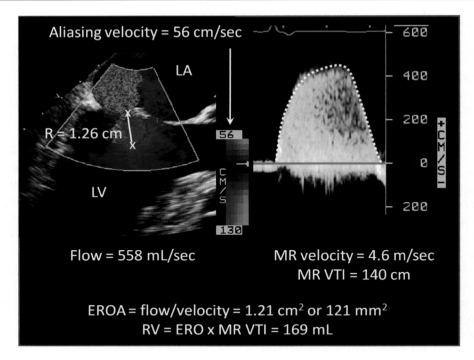

Fig. 3.2 Assessment of MR severity using the flow convergence or proximal isovelocity surface area (PISA) method. To calculate the flow rate across the regurgitant orifice, the baseline of the color scale has been shifted up to decrease the aliasing velocity to 56 cm/s (velocity at the *blue-red* border), which allows the flow convergence (*blue*) to be seen. The radius (*r*) of the flow convergence is used in the formula for calculation of the instantaneous regurgitant flow: flow rate = $2 \times \pi \times r^2 \times V_{aliasing}$. In this example, flow rate is 556 mL/s. Division of this value by the jet velocity allows calculation of the effective regurgitant orifice of mitral regurgitation. The orifice area is then multiplied by the time–velocity integral of the regurgitant jet to obtain the regurgitant volume. A=left atrium. LV=left ventricle

Quantitative measurements of the RV can be obtained using either the *pulsed-wave Doppler* method or the Proximal Isovelocity Surface Area (*PISA*) method. The pulsed-wave Doppler method requires calculation of the aortic and mitral stroke volumes. In the absence of aortic regurgitation, the difference between these two stroke volumes should equal the RV.

The PISA method is based on the law of conservation of mass. Briefly, as the regurgitant flow approaches the regurgitant orifice, it progressively accelerates and converges on the orifice in hemispheric layers of equal velocity. Because the volume flow that streams across any of these concentric isovelocity shells equals the volume flow that crosses the regurgitant orifice, it is possible to calculate the regurgitant orifice area using the continuity equation. One simply needs to measure the radius of the hemispheric flow convergence shell, the velocity of blood at the same level, and the velocity of blood in the regurgitant orifice. Using color flow mapping, the two first parameters can be easily obtained, the radius of the isovelocity shell corresponding to the distance separating the orifice from red-blue or blue-red color transition at the aliasing velocity and velocity of blood across that hemispheric shell corresponding to the aliasing velocity, which is always displayed on the screen of the ultrasound system. Once the EROA has been measured, one simply needs to multiply it by the time-velocity integral of the regurgitant flow (using CW-Doppler) to obtain the RV (Fig. 3.2). Values >60 mL, for the RV, and ≥40 mm,[2] for the EROA, indicate severe MR.

Etiology

Transthoracic echocardiography (TTE) allows for the accurate determination of the cause of MR (Fig. 3.3). Gray-scale echocardiography frequently permits identification of the underlying cause of the regurgitation,

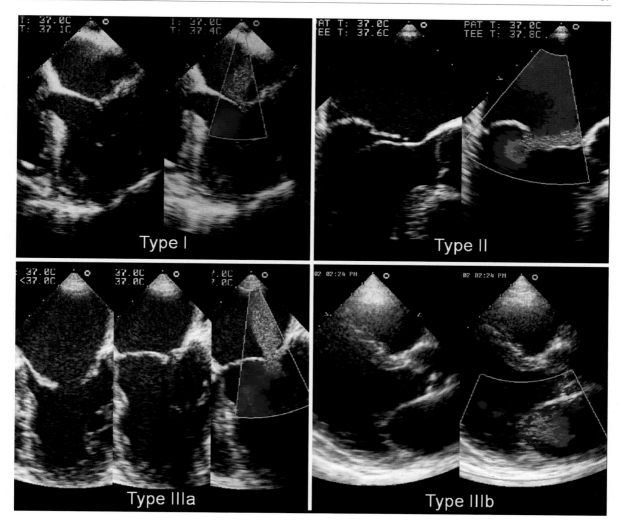

Fig. 3.3 Representative transesophageal or transthoracic echocardiographic still frames showing the various mechanisms of mitral regurgitation. *Type I*: an example of isolated anular dilatation leading to moderate MR. Both mitral leaflets are normal in appearance and motion. Coaptation length is short. The regurgitant jet has a typical central orientation. *Type II*: an example of flail posterior leaflet with the tip of the leaflet overriding the mitral annulus and floating in the left atrium. A ruptured chord is attached to the free edge the flail leaflet. The regurgitant jet is typically eccentric and oriented at the opposite of the prolapsed leaflet. *Type IIIa*: an example of rheumatic mitral regurgitation. The mitral leaflets are thickened, and the valve has a characteristic restrictive opening. There is a central lack of coaptation, resulting in a central jet of MR. *Type IIIb*: an example of ischemic mitral regurgitation. Strut chordae to the anterior and posterior leaflets exert an abnormal traction on the body of the leaflets, which displaces the leaflets towards the ventricular apex, creating an area of tenting above the mitral annulus and an incomplete coaptation.

such as rupture of chordae tendinae, mitral valve prolapse with or without a flail leaflet, rheumatic mitral disease, vegetations, and LV dilatation. It may also show calcification of the posterior mitral annulus. This technique is also useful for estimating LV end-diastolic and end-systolic volumes and ejection fraction. Color Doppler is also commonly used for the detection and also the characterization of MR. The direction of the MR jet provides valuable information on the etiology of MR. Eccentric jets, which are easily identifiable using Color Doppler, are indeed frequently associated with an opposing leaflet prolapse. In case of nondiagnostic TTE or prior to mitral valve surgery, transesophageal echocardiography (TEE) can also be useful. When compared to surgical diagnosis, the accuracy of TEE is 99% for etiology, mechanism, presence of vegetations, prolapsed or flail segment, and 88% for ruptured chordae. Diagnostic accuracy is higher for TEE than for TTE.[21] Finally, 3D-echocardiography is a promising new tool for assessing the mitral valve but remains under evaluation.

Repairability

Mitral valve prolapse is associated with a 90% probability of surgical repair, as compared to 63% in case of rheumatic fever.[21] As echocardiography allows for a precise description of the etiology of MR, it also allows for the prediction of valve repairability.

Cardiac Catheterization

With the advent of echocardiography, invasive cardiac catheterization is seldom useful unless discrepancies are found between symptoms and echocardiography.[12] However, performance of a coronary angiogram remains recommended prior to mitral valve surgery to assess the presence of coronary artery disease. In the near future, computerized tomography could become an interesting alternative to conventional coronary angiography in this indication, particularly in patients with a low probability of coronary artery disease.[23]

Natural History

The natural history of chronic MR is highly variable, depending on the volume of regurgitation, the LV function, and the underlying cause of MR. Currently, most of the data available on the natural history of MR have been obtained in patients with flail leaflets. These observations may thus not be pertinent to MR of other causes.

Chronic severe MR is associated with a 10% per year risk of major complications, which include congestive heart failure, infective endocarditis, cerebrovascular events due to LA enlargement and development of AF, need for mitral valve surgery, and death.[24,25] Several prognostic factors have been identified in cohort studies.[26–30]

As demonstrated by Ling et al.,[31] overall survival is influenced by the presence of symptoms and LV systolic dysfunction. Patients in NYHA functional class III or IV entail a much higher mortality rate (34.0% yearly) than those in class I or II (4.1% yearly, $p < 0.001$). Similarly, patients with reduced LVEF (<60%) exhibit a poorer 10-year overall survival (42% ± 12%) than patients with a normal LVEF (>60%, 61% ± 4%, $p = 0.034$).

The occurrence of AF is also associated with a poorer survival. The annual incidence of AF is estimated at 5% per year.[29] At 10 years, the incidence is higher in patients with LA enlargement (defined as an LA size > 50 mm), and in patients older than 65 years.[29] Finally, the presence of PHT (defined as a pulmonary artery systolic pressure >50 mmHg at rest or >60 mmHg during exercise) is also associated with reduced survival.[32]

Recently, Enriquez-Sarano et al.[33] have shown that the overall survival was directly and independently related to the severity of MR, as measured by the EROA. These authors studied the outcomes of 456 patients with severe isolated MR and observed that 5-year overall survival was better (91% ± 3%) in patients with an EROA <20 mm,[2] than in those with an EROA ≥40 mm^2 (58% ± 9%).

The yearly incidence of *sudden cardiac death* (SCD) approaches 1.8%.[34] It is higher in patients in NYHA class III/IV (7.8%/year) than in those in NYHA class II (3.1%/year) or NYHA class I (1.0%/year).[35] It is also more frequent in the presence of LV dysfunction (12.7%/year when LVEF is <50% versus <1.5%/year when LVEF is >50%). Other risk factors for SCD include a history of syncope or near syncope, a prolonged QT interval, inferolateral repolarization abnormalities, frequent or complex ventricular premature beats, and prolapse of both the anterior and posterior mitral leaflets.[36–38]

Indications for Mitral Valve Surgery

The only effective treatment of chronic severe MR is surgical repair or replacement of the mitral valve. The indications for surgery are based on natural history data. The medical treatment is limited to the management of heart failure (ACE inhibitors, diuretics) and AF (anticoagulation). Prevention of bacterial endocarditis is no longer recommended.

The optimal timing of corrective surgery is determined by the severity of MR, the presence of symptoms, the LV systolic function, the feasibility of valve repair, the presence of AF, the presence of PHT, and finally the preference and expectations of the patient.[20,39]

The presence of symptoms is a class I indication for corrective surgery in patients with severe chronic MR (ESC and ACC/AHA Guidelines: class IB). Delaying surgery until moderate to severe symptoms occur is associated with an increased operative (6.7% in NYHA IV patients, 2.2% in NYHA III patients, and 1.2% in NYHA I-II patients) and long-term mortality (48% versus 76%).[40] Symptomatic patients with an LVEF below 30% should, nonetheless, be considered at high operative risk, especially if valve replacement is necessary. In such patients, medical management may be preferable. In patients who do not respond to medical therapy, surgical intervention may be considered if the mitral annular–papillary muscle continuity can be maintained either by valve repair or replacement with preservation of the chordal apparatus (ESC and ACC/AHA Guidelines: class IIA).

In asymptomatic patients, mitral surgery is indicated when *LVEF is <60%, LV end-systolic LV diameter is >40 mm or both* (both ESC and ACC/AHA Guidelines: class IB), as in these patients 10-year postoperative survival is at least 20% lower than in patients with an LVEF >60%.[41–43]

In asymptomatic patients with a normal LVEF, mitral surgery is also recommended in the *presence of AF or PHT*.

In asymptomatic patients with severe chronic MR, a normal LV systolic function, no AF or PHT, the ESC guidelines recommend a watchfulwaiting approach.[39,44] These patients should be serially followed-up every 6 to 12 months or sooner if symptoms occur, using TTE. The AHA/ACC guidelines take a more aggressive approach, recommending to proceed to surgery in the absence of any MR-related complications, if mitral valve repair can be performed with a likelihood of >90%, and a very low operative mortality. In these patients, mitral repair can be proposed whenever the EROA exceeds 40 mm² and the mitral valve is repairable.[33] Recently published propensity score-based comparisons between early surgical and watchful waiting strategies support this more aggressive attitude (Fig. 3.4).[45,46]

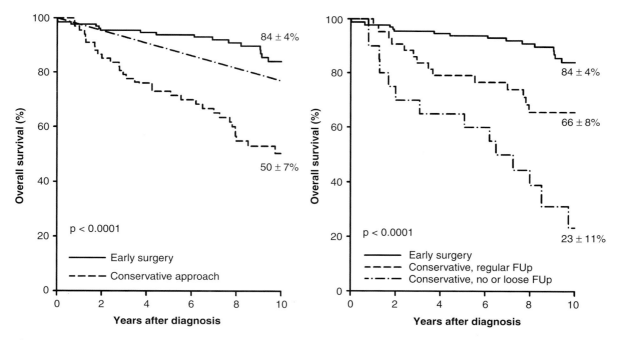

Fig. 3.4 *Left panel*: Kaplan–Meier curves for overall survival comparing patients undergoing early surgery (*solid line*), those treated conservatively (*dashed line*) and the age- and gender matched Belgian population (*dashed dotted line*). *Right panel*: Kaplan–Meier curves for overall survival compared for patients undergoing early surgery (*solid line*), those treated conservatively and being followed-up regularly (*dashed line*) or those treated conservatively and undergoing a looser follow-up (*dashed dotted line*) (Adapted from Montant et al.[46]; used with permission)

Surgical Considerations

Valve repair and valve replacement are the two available surgical procedures for the treatment of chronic MR. The choice of procedure depends mainly upon the anatomy of the valve (repairability) and the skills of the surgical team. Besides indications for surgery previously discussed, it is important to stratify the surgical risk of each patient. The reference risk stratification for mitral surgery is based on the data of the Society of Cardiothoracic Surgeons of Great Britain and Ireland.[47]

Whenever feasible, *mitral valve repair* is the preferred surgical treatment for MR as it is associated with a very lower operative mortality, particularly in asymptomatic individuals aged 65 years or less, and a better overall survival at 10 years (68% versus 52%) than mitral valve replacement.[48–55] Overall, 5-and 10-year mortality rates after mitral valve repair are similar to the expected mortality rates in a normal age-matched population (13.5% and 28.4%, respectively).[48]

When mitral repair is not feasible, *bioprosthetic or mechanical valve replacement* should be proposed. In all cases, the subvalvular apparatus should be conserved in order to preserve left ventricular geometry and function.[56] Bioprosthetic and mechanical valves expose the patients to different prosthetic-related complications, i.e., thromboembolic complications with mechanical valves and structural valve deterioration with bioprostheses.[57–59] Bioprosthetic valves should be recommended in patients in whom oral anticoagulants are contraindicated and in those aged 65 years or more, as the risk of bioprosthetic structural deterioration is less in elderly people. There are few randomized comparisons between mechanical valves and bioprostheses. In the Veterans Affairs randomized trial, 181 patients were randomized to receive the Hancock bioprosthetic valve or the Bjork-Shiley mechanical valve.[57] After a 15-year follow-up, all-cause mortality was similar in both treatment groups (81% versus 79%). Primary valve failure was more common in patients aged 65 years or less who received a bioprosthesis (44% versus 4%). On the other hand, bleeding complications were more frequent in patients who received a mechanical prosthesis.

Percutaneous mitral valve repair is currently under study.[60,61] Several devices are currently being investigated. The only preliminary results available are from the Everest trial, in which percutaneous mitral valve repair was performed using a clip device.[62] The results indicate that approximately than half of the patients still have 2+ or more MR at 6 months. At this stage, percutaneous valve repair can only be recommended to patients in whom surgery cannot be performed at acceptable risks.

References

1. Perloff JK, Roberts WC. The mitral apparatus – functional anatomy of mitral regurgitation. *Circulation*. 1972;46:227-239.
2. Carpentier AF, Lessana A, Relland J, et al. The "Physio-Ring": an advanced concept in mitral valve annuloplasty. *Ann Thorac Surg*. 1995;60:1177-1186.
3. Lam JHC, Ranganathan N, Wigle ED, Silver MD. Morphology of the human heart valve I. Chordae tendinae: a new classification. *Circulation*. 1970;41:449-458.
4. Rusted IE, Schiefly CH, Edwards JE. Studies of the mitral valve. I. Anatomical features of the normal mitral valve and associated structures. *Circulation*. 1952;6:825-831.
5. Voci P, Bilotta F, Caretta Q, Mercanti C, Marino B. Papillary muscle perfusion pattern: a hypothesis for ischemic papillary muscle dysfunction. *Circulation*. 1995;91:1714-1718.
6. Carpentier A. Cardiac valve surgery – the "French" correction. *J Thorac Cardiovasc Surg*. 1983;86:323-337.
7. Schwammenthal E, Chen C, Benning E, Block E, Breithardt G, Levine RA. Dynamics of mitral regurgitant flow and orifice area: physiologic application of the proximal flow convergence method. *Circulation*. 1994;90:307-322.
8. Gaasch W, Meyer T. Left ventricular response to mitral regurgitation: implications for management. *Circulation*. 2008;118:2298-2303.
9. Janicki JS, Brower GL, Gardner JD, et al. Cardiac mast cell regulation of matrix metalloproteinase-related ventricular remodeling in chronic pressure or volume overload. *Cardiovasc Res*. 2006;69:657-665.
10. Grossman W, Jones D, McLaurin LP. Wall stress and patterns of hypertrophy in the human left ventricule. *J Clin Invest*. 1975;56:56-64.
11. Carabello BA. Mitral regurgitation: basic pathophysiologic principles. *Mod Concepts Cardiovasc Dis*. 1988;57:53-58.
12. Detaint D, Messika-Zeitoun D, Avierinos JF, et al. B-Type Natriuretic Peptide in organic mitral regurgitation. Determinants and impact on outcome. *Circulation*. 2005; 111:2391-2397.
13. Enriquez-Sarano M, Basmadjian AJ, Rossi A. Progression of mitral regurgitation: a prospective Doppler echocardiographic study. *J Am Coll Cardiol*. 1999;34:1137-1144.
14. Iung B, Baron G, Butchaert EG, et al. A prospective survey of patients with valvular heart disease: the euro heart survey on valvular heart disease. *Eur Heart J*. 2003;24:1231-1243.
15. Singh JP, Evans JC, Levy D, et al. Prevalence and clinical determinants of mitral, tricuspid and aortic regurgitation. *Am J Cardiol*. 1999;83:897-902.
16. Jones EC, Devereux RB, Roman MJ, et al. Prevalence and correlates of mitral regurgitation in a population-based

sample (the Strong Heart study). *Am J Cardiol*. 2001; 87:298-304.

17. Flack JM, Kvasnicka JH, Gardin JM, et al. Anthropometric and physiologic correlates of mitral valve prolapse in a biethnic cohort of young adults: the CARDIA study. *Am Heart J*. 1999;138:486-492.

18. Freed LA, Levy D, Levine RA, et al. Prevalence and clinical outcome of mitral valve prolapse. *N Engl J Med*. 1999; 341:1-7.

19. Desjardins VA, Enriquez-Sarano M, Tajik AJ, et al. Intensity of murmurs correlates with severity of valvular regurgitation. *Am J Med*. 1996;100:149-156.

20. Bonow RO, Carabello BA, Chatterjee K, et al. ACC/AHA 2006 guidelines for the management of patients with valvular heart disease. A report of the American College of Cardiology/American Heart Association Task Force on Practice Guidelines. *J Am Coll Cardiol*. 2006;48:e1.

21. Enriquez-Sarano M, Freeman WK, Tribouilloy CM, et al. Functional anatomy of mitral regurgitation: accuracy and outcome implications of transoesophageal echocardiography. *J Am Coll Cardiol*. 1999;34:1129-1136.

22. Zoghbi WA, Enriquez-Sarano M, Foster E, et al. American Society of Echocardiography. Recommendations for evaluation of the severity of native valvular regurgitation with two-dimensional and Doppler echocardiography. *J Am Soc Echocardiogr*. 2003;16:777-802.

23. Pouleur AC, le Polain de Waroux JB, et al. Usefulness of 40-slice multidetector row computed tomography to detect coronary disease in patients prior to cardiac valve surgery. *Eur Radiol*. 2007;17:3199-207.

24. Allen H, Harris A, Leatham A. Significance and prognosis of an isolated late systolic murmur: a 9 to 22 year follow up. *Br Heart J*. 1974;36:525-532.

25. Mills P, Rose J, Hollingsworth J, et al. Long-term prognosis of mitral-valve prolapse. *N Engl J Med*. 1977;297:13-18.

26. Avierinos JF, Gersh BJ, Melton LJ, et al. Natural history of asymptomatic mitral valve prolapse in the community. *Circulation*. 2002;106:1355-1361.

27. Zuppiroli A, Rinaldi M, Kramer-Fox R, et al. Natural history of mitral valve prolapse. *Am J Cardiol*. 1995;75:1028-1032.

28. Kim S, Kuroda T, Nishinaga M, et al. Relationship between severity of mitral regurgitation and prognosis of mitral valve prolapse: echocardiographic follow-up study. *Am Heart J*. 1996;132:348-355.

29. Grigioni F, Avierinos JF, Ling LH, et al. Atrial fibrillation complicating the course of degenerative mitral regurgitation: determinants and long-term outcome. *J Am Coll Cardiol*. 2002;40:84-92.

30. Ling LH, Enriquez-Sarano M, Seward JB, et al. Early surgery in patients with mitral regurgitation due to flail leaflets. A long-term outcome study. *Circulation*. 1997;96:1819-1825.

31. Ling LH, Enriquez-Sarano M, Seward JB, et al. Clinical outcome of mitral regurgitation due to flail leaflet. *N Engl J Med*. 1996;335:1417-1423.

32. Tanaka K, Ohtaki E, Matsumura T, et al. Impact of a preoperative mitral regurgitation scoring system on outcome of surgical repair for mitral valve prolapse. *Am J Cardiol*. 2003;92:1306-1309.

33. Enriquez-Sarano M, Avierinos JF, Messika-Zeitoun D, et al. Quantitative determinants of the outcome of asymptomatic mitral regurgitation. *N Engl J Med*. 2005;352:875-883.

34. Boudoulas H, Schaal SF, Stang JM, et al. Mitral valve prolapse: cardiac arrest with long-term survival. *Int J Cardiol*. 1990;26:37-44.

35. Grigioni F, Enriquez-Sarano M, Ling LH, et al. Sudden death due to mitral regurgitation due to flail leaflet. *J Am Coll Cardiol*. 1999;34:2078-2085.

36. Kligfield P, Levy D, Devereux RB, et al. Arrhythmias and sudden death in mitral valve prolapse. *Am Heart J*. 1987; 113:1298-1307.

37. Kligfield P, Devereux RB. Is the mitral valve prolapse patient at high risk of sudden death identifiable? *Cardiovasc Clin*. 1990;21:143-157.

38. Alpert JS. Association between arrhythmias and mitral valve prolapse. *Arch Intern Med*. 1984;144:2333-2334.

39. Vahanian A, Baumgartner H, Bax J, et al. Guidelines on the management of valvular heart disease: The Task Force on the Management of Valvular Heart Disease of the European Society of Cardiology. *Eur Heart J*. 2007;28:230-268.

40. Tribouilloy CM, Enriquez-Sarano M, Schaff HV, et al. Impact of preoperative symptoms on survival after surgical correction of organic mitral regurgitation: rationale for optimizing surgical indications. *Circulation*. 1999;99:400-405.

41. Enriquez-Sarano M, Tajik AJ, Schaff HV, et al. Echocardiographic prediction of survival after surgical correction of organic mitral regurgitation. *Circulation*. 1994; 90:830-837.

42. STS database 1997.

43. Savage EB, Ferguson TB, DiSesa VJ. Use of mitral valve repair: analysis of contemporary United States experience reported to the Society of Thoracic Surgeons National Cardiac Database. *Ann Thorac Surg*. 2007;31: 267-275.

44. Rosenhek R, Rader F, Klaar U, et al. Outcome of watchful waiting in asymptomatic severe mitral regurgitation. *Circulation*. 2006;113:2238-2244.

45. Kang DH, Kim JH, Rim JH, et al. Comparison of early surgery versus conventional treatment in asymptomatic severe mitral regurgitation. *Circulation*. 2009;119:797-804.

46. Montant P, Chenot F, Robert A, et al. Long-term survival in asymptomatic patients with severe degenerative mitral regurgitation. A propensity score based comparison between an "early surgical" and a "conservative" treatment approach. *J Thorac Cardiovasc Surg*. 2009;138:1339-1348.

47. Ambler G, Omar RZ, Royston P, et al. Generic, simple risk stratification model for heart valve surgery. *Circulation*. 2005;112:224-231.

48. Suri RM, Schaff HV, Dearani JA, et al. Survival advantage and improved durability of mitral repair for leaflet prolapse subsets in the current era. *Ann Thorac Surg*. 2006;82:819-826.

49. Enriquez-Sarano M, Schaff HV, Orszulak TA, et al. Valve repair improves the outcome of surgery for mitral regurgitation. *Circulation*. 1995;91:1022-1028.

50. Galloway AC, Colvin SB, Baumann FG, et al. Current concepts of mitral valve reconstruction for mitral insufficiency. *Circulation*. 1988;78:1087-1098.

51. Lee EM, Shapiro LM, Wells FC. Superiority of mitral valve repair in surgery for degenerative mitral regurgitation. *Eur Heart J*. 1997;18:655-663.

52. Yau TM, El-Ghoneimi YA, Armstrong S, et al. Mitral valve repair and replacement for rheumatic disease. *J Thorac Cardiovasc Surg*. 2000;119:53-60.

53. Mohty D, Orszulak TA, Schaff HV, et al. Very long-term survival and durability of mitral valve repair for mitral valve prolapse. *Circulation*. 2001;104:I1-I7.

54. Thourani VH, Weintraub WS, Guyton RA, et al. Outcomes and long-term survival for patients undergoing mitral valve repair versus replacement: effect of age and concomitant coronary artery bypass grafting. *Circulation*. 2003; 108:298-304.

55. Moss RR, Humphries KH, Gao M, et al. Outcome of mitral valve repair or replacement: a comparison by propensity score analysis. *Circulation*. 2003;108(Suppl 1):II90.

56. Rozich JD, Carabello BA, Usher BW, et al. Mitral valve replacement with and without chordal preservation in patients with chronic mitral regurgitation. *Circulation*. 1992; 86:1718-1726.

57. Hammermeister KE, Sethi GK, Henderson WG, et al. A comparison of outcomes in men 11 years after heart-valve replacement with a mechanical valve or bioprosthesis: Veterans Affairs Cooperative Study on Valvular Heart Disease. *N Engl J Med*. 1993;328:1289-1296.

58. Hammermeister K, Sethi GK, Henderson WG, et al. Outcomes 15 years after valve replacement with a mechanical versus a bioprosthetic valve: final report of the Veterans Affairs randomized trial. *J Am Coll Cardiol*. 2000;36: 1152-1158.

59. Grunkemeier GL, Starr A, Rahimtoola SH. Prosthetic heart valve performance: long-term follow-up. *Curr Probl Cardiol*. 1992;17:329-406.

60. Block PC. Percutaneous mitral valve repair: are they changing the guard? *Circulation*. 2005;111:2154-2156.

61. Daimon M, Shiota T, Gillinov AM, et al. Percutaneous mitral valve repair for chronic ischemic mitral regurgitation: a real-time three-dimensional echocardiographic study in an ovine model. *Circulation*. 2005;111:2183-2189.

62. Feldman T, Wasserman HS, Herrmann HC, et al. Percutaneous mitral valve repair using the edge-to-edge technique six-month results of the EVEREST phase I clinical trial. *J Am Coll Cardiol*. 2005;46:2134-2140.

Chronic Ischemic Mitral Regurgitation

4

Jean-Louis Vanoverschelde, Gébrine El Khoury,
and Agnès Pasquet

Introduction

Ischemic mitral regurgitation (MR) is mitral regurgitation due to complications of coronary artery disease, in particular myocardial infarction (MI), and not the fortuitous association of coronary artery disease with intrinsic valve disease such as degenerative, myxomatous, and connective tissue valvular disease, spontaneous ruptured chordae tendinae, and other causes of acute or chronic MR due to infection, inflammation, trauma, congenital abnormalities (including mitral valve (MV) prolapse), annular calcification, or tumor. Accordingly, the term ischemic MR should be restricted to chronic MR, occurring more than 2 weeks after MI and in the absence of structural MV disease. From a pathogenic point of view, it is a manifestation of postinfarction ventricular remodeling. The size, location, and transmurality of the MI sets in motion left ventricle (LV) remodeling that determines the severity, time course, and clinical manifestation of ischemic MR. The presentation develops insidiously over time in association with congestive heart failure.

Prevalence and Prognostic Impact

The prevalence of ischemic MR varies according to the technique used for its detection. Between 17% and 55% of patients develop a mitral systolic murmur or echocardiographic evidence of ischemic MR early after acute MI (AMI).[1-4] In patients undergoing cardiac catheterization within 6 h of the onset of their AMI, 18% have ventriculographic evidence of ischemic MR, and in 3%, the degree of MR is severe.[5] In a large study of patients undergoing elective cardiac catheterization for symptomatic coronary artery disease, 19% had ventriculographic evidence of MR.[6] In most of these patients, the degree of MR was mild, but in 7% of them, the degree of MR was 2+ or greater, and in 3%, MR was severe with evidence of heart failure.[6]

These data indicate that ischemic MR is frequent early after AMI, but in many patients it is mild or disappears completely. The relatively high incidence of ischemic MR (11–19%) in catheterized patients with symptomatic coronary artery disease suggests that chronic ischemic MR persists in many patients after acute infarction and may subsequently develop in others.

The presence of chronic ischemic MR carries an increased risk of heart failure and death, which is independent of LV systolic function. Importantly, a graded positive association between the severity of MR and risk of death and heart failure has been evidenced. Even moderate degrees of MR, as evaluated by the proximal isovelocity surface area (PISA) method, carry a negative prognostic impact, patients with an effective regurgitant orifice area (EROA) >20 mm² having a threefold risk to develop heart failure and a twofold risk of dying within the next 5 years.[7]

Mechanisms of Ischemic MR

Although chronic ischemic MR may occasionally result from papillary muscle elongation and subsequent MV prolapse, the vast majority have incomplete

J.-L. Vanoverschelde (✉)
Pôle de Recherche Cardiovasculaire, Institut de Recherche Expérimentale et Clinique, Université catholique de Louvain, Brussels, Belgium
e-mail: jean-louis.vanoverschelde@uclouvain.be

R.S. Bonser et al. (eds.), *Mitral Valve Surgery*,
DOI: 10.1007/978-1-84996-426-5_4, © Springer-Verlag London Limited 2011

MV closure due to papillary muscle and chordal restriction of leaflet motion.[8] Pathologic studies consistently show fibrosis and atrophy of infarcted papillary muscles, and none demonstrate chordal elongation.[9,10] Nevertheless, surgeons describe elongated chordae in some patients with MI and MR.[11,12] In those patients, elongated chordae and MV prolapse without MR probably antedate the infarction. In a patient with pre-existing MV prolapse, MI may cause the previously competent valve to leak. This hypothesis explains sporadic observations of MV prolapse in patients with chronic ischemic MR, but needs pre-infarction echocardiograms for confirmation.

The mechanism of ischemic MR requires a combination of reduced LV closing forces and leaflet tethering, the effects of which are amplified in the setting of annular dilatation.[8]

Impaired Contractile Function

Although impairment of LV contractile function contributes to the development of ischemic MR, it is unusual for LV dysfunction to cause MR in the absence of LV remodeling. In patients with ischemic MR, changes in LV contractile function over time affect the severity of MR.[8,13,14] Treatments that influence LV closing forces, such as revascularization,[15,16] cardiac resynchronization therapy (CRT),[17,18] and medical therapy,[19–21] may significantly modulate ischemic MR. The contribution of LV dyssynchrony, and particularly papillary muscle dyssynchrony, has been more recently recognized. In patients with left bundle branch block, mechanical activation occurs first in the segments adjacent to the posterior papillary muscle and is delayed in the segments adjacent to the anterolateral papillary muscle. The interpapillary muscle activation time delay varies substantially from patient to patient and is significantly correlated with the severity of MR.[18] With CRT, this inter-papillary activation delay is shortened and its changes correlate well with reduction of MR.

Increased Leaflet Tethering

The prerequisite for the initial development of MR is the presence of local or global LV remodeling, causing alteration in the geometrical relationship between the LV and valve apparatus and generating a restricted leaflet motion, termed "incomplete mitral leaflet closure."[8,14,22] In systole, the mitral leaflets normally come together near the level of their annular insertions, their chordal attachments to the papillary muscles preventing them from prolapsing into the left atrium (LA). In ischemic MR, the leaflet attachments are displaced apically and outward, restricting their movement during coaptation.[23]

In the classical form of ischemic MR, which involves a posterior wall motion abnormality with regional remodeling, the infero-posterior wall bulges outward, leading to the posterolateral and apical displacement of the posterior papillary muscle (Fig. 4.1).[24,25] As the papillary muscle contributes chordae to both leaflets, the

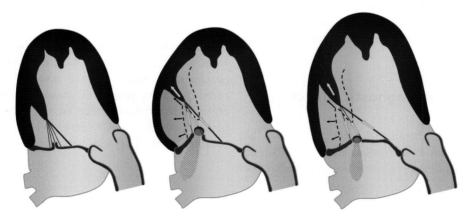

Fig. 4.1 *Left panel*: Normal coaptation of mitral leaflets. *Middle panel*: Typical asymmetric tenting of the mitral valve as seen in patients with inferior-posterior myocardial infarction. Both leaflets are posteriorly displaced, resulting in the appearance of prevalent restriction of posterior leaflet. The basal anterior leaflet is also tethered, but distal to the strut chordae is less restricted than the posterior one. The MR jet is usually eccentric and oriented towards the posterior wall of the left atrium. *Right panel*: Symmetrical tenting of the mitral leaflets due to the predominant apical displacement of both leaflets as can be seen after an anterior myocardial infarction. The MR jet is usually central. Ao: aorta, LA : left atrium, LV : left ventricle

posterior commissure and the posterior aspects of both mitral leaflets become displaced apically and posteriorly.[23] The posterior leaflet is usually drawn more posteriorly than apically (more parallel to the posterior wall), preventing it from reaching its normal, more anteriorly located coaptation point. Accordingly, the coaptation point moves posteriorly, creating the asymmetric tethering shape. The anterior leaflet is also often tethered, albeit to a lesser extent than the posterior leaflet. Restriction of the anterior leaflet mainly arises from the tethered secondary chordae, which exert forces at the body of the anterior leaflet and produce a typical bending in the middle of this leaflet, which is sometimes referred to as the "hockey stick configuration".[24,26] As a consequence, the posterior aspect of the anterior leaflet overrides that of the posterior leaflet, leading to a posteriorly oriented MR jet.[24] Depending on the extent of the tethering process of the posterior leaflet, the jet can be either centrally and posteriorly directed, when the tethering effect involves a large part of the posterior leaflet, or follow the coaptation line, when the tethering effect involves predominantly the medial commissure.

In the global form of ischemic MR (Fig. 4.1), which resembles that seen in dilated cardiomyopathy, the coaptation line of the MV is moved apically, with a large symmetrical tenting area. In these cases, both leaflets are involved to a similar degree, the MR jet originates from the entire coaptation line and is centrally oriented. This form of ischemic MR is typically associated with large anterior infarctions or multiple infarctions. Global enlargement of the LV usually occurs in association with increased sphericity and annular dilatation.[24,25]

Annular Dilatation

The normal mitral annulus typically presents a saddle shape that is accentuated during systole to reduce the stress on the valve components.[27] In patients with ischemic MR, the annulus is often dilated and flattened with loss of the saddle shape.[28] Loss of the saddle shape reduces leaflet curvature and increases leaflet stress. The annulus usually dilates more along its inferior-posterior aspects (Fig. 4.2). The anterior and posterior portions and inter-trigonal distance dilate proportionally.[29] Finally, the annular area change, an index of the sphincteric function, and the annular motion are decreased in these patients indicating a loss of annular contraction.[30]

Annular dilation generally acts as a modulating factor because it is able to increase significantly the degree of MR in the presence of leaflet tethering. In the absence of leaflet tethering, isolated annular dilatation rarely causes significant degrees of MR. Indeed, in patients with lone atrial fibrillation, who develop mitral annular dilation in the absence of ventricular abnormalities,

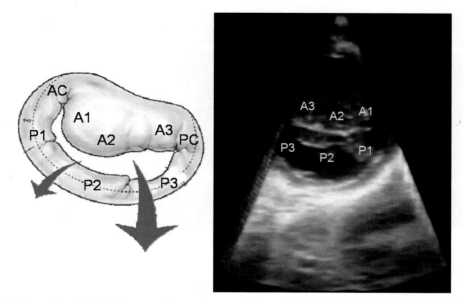

Fig. 4.2 Typical deformation of the inferior posterior annulus as seen from the LA (surgical view on the left panel) and from the LV cavity (with 3D echocardiography on the right panel)

MR is rarely of significant importance.[31] Annular dilatation, thus appears to play an adjunctive role, with evidence that it increases MR at different levels of papillary muscle displacement.[8,32]

Dynamic Nature of Ischemic MR

Chronic ischemic MR is a dynamic phenomenon and its severity varies greatly over time. This characteristic depends on the dynamic interplay between tethering and closing forces, and on the physiologic and pharmacologic factors able to modify this equilibrium. Typical examples of this phenomenon are the dramatic effects of inotropic agents and anesthetic induction on intraoperative evaluation of the severity of MR.[19–21] The inotropic agents (i.e., dobutamine infusion) increase dP/dt and thereby the closing forces reducing

MR.[20] The general anesthesia usually reduces LV preload, which in turn decreases ventricular size and the tethering forces and consequently reduces the MR severity.[21] The same effect is obtained with diuretic therapy.

Chronic ischemic MR is also very sensitive to exercise (Fig. 4.3).[33,34] The increase in MR during exercise depends directly on exercise-induced changes in mitral deformation indexes (systolic annular area and tenting area), and local remodeling of the part of the LV supporting the posterior papillary muscle, whereas it is inversely related to the presence of contractile reserve and independent of the degree of MR at rest. Therefore, exercise is utilized as stressor to unmask the dynamic component of chronic ischemic MR during stress echocardiography in patients with heart failure. Changes in regurgitant volume (RV) during exercise have been shown to be the main driver of the exercise-induced changes in forward stroke volume, capillary wedge pressure, and exercise capacity in patients with heart failure.[33]

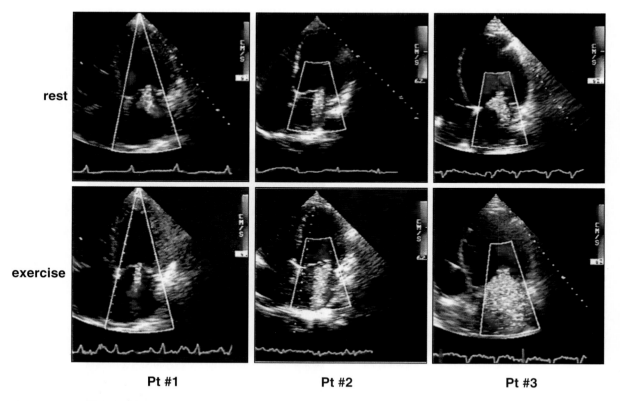

Fig. 4.3 Representative echocardiographic examples of dynamic changes in severity of ischemic MR during exercise in three patients with ischemic heart failure symptoms (Adapted from Lapu-Bula et al.,[33] used with permission)

Evaluation of Patients with Ischemic MR

Evaluation of patients with ischemic MR requires a multi-disciplinary and often a multi-modality approach.

Echocardiography

Echocardiography is essential for establishing the presence of MR, quantitating its severity and hemodynamic consequences, and ascertaining its ischemic origin. As for nonischemic forms of MR, grading of the severity of ischemic MR requires an integrated approach that includes assessment of valve morphology, the size of the regurgitant jet in the LA, the proximal regurgitant jet width or vena contracta, the pulmonary venous flow pattern, and the measurement of the EROA and the RV.[35]

Quantitative parameters of MR severity can be obtained using either the PISA or the Doppler methods. Caution should, nonetheless, be exercised when using the PISA method for assessing MR severity. First, recent studies have shown that the shape of the flow convergence zone is rarely hemispherical in patients with ischemic MR, which frequently leads to underestimation of the EROA and the RV by this method.[36,37] Second, the severity of ischemic MR greatly varies during systole, being the greatest at the beginning and end of systole and least in mid-systole; when the LV pressure is maximal, LV volume is reduced and the mitral leaflets are pushed back into the annular plane.[38] This phenomenon has important implications with respect to the use of EROA as an index of MR, implying that this should be averaged through systole.[39] The use of volumetric methods for calculating RV may thus be preferable in patients with ischemic MR.

Echocardiography is also useful to evaluate the characteristics of the LV, particularly its volumes, its sphericity index, its ejection fraction, its diastolic function, and the distribution of its wall motion abnormalities. It also allows making several anatomic measurements that reflect the pathophysiology of ischemic MR, including the tenting area,[23] the leaflet angles,[40] the coaptation depth,[23,33] the bending distance, and the leaflet length (Fig. 4.4). These measurements

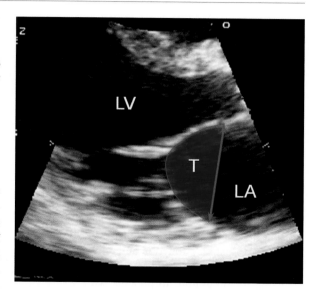

Fig. 4.4 Parasternal long-axis view of the left ventricle (LV), and left atrium (LA) demonstrating systolic apical displacement of mitral valve leaflets into LV with large tenting area (T). Note that these deformations result in lack of central coaptation between anterior and posterior leaflets. *Arrows* indicate position of mitral annulus plane

should be made in the parasternal long-axis view in mid-systole. In normal individuals, the coaptation depth and the tenting area does not exceed 0.6 cm and 1 cm² respectively.[24] Greater degrees of morphologic disturbance have been shown to be predictive of the likelihood of MR persistence following mitral annuloplasty, with the optimal cut-offs for distinguishing patients with persistent MR being a coaptation depth >0.6 cm, a tenting area of >2.5 cm², or a posterior leaflet angle >45°. Recently, the tenting volume derived from 3D-echocardiography has been shown to be a better index of MV remodeling than the 2D tenting area.[41]

Stress Echocardiography

Exercise echocardiography can be used to evaluate the dynamic nature of ischemic MR.[33,34] Changes in EROA exceeding 13 mm² have been shown to carry adverse prognostic implications and to predict the occurrence of both heart failure and death.[42] Dobutamine echocardiography can also be used to evaluate myocardial viability.[43] The absence of myocardial viability or contractile reserve seems to be an independent predictor of a poor outcome in patients undergoing mitral annuloplasty.[44] On the other hand, reliable improvement in moderate ischemic MR by isolated coronary artery bypass graft (CABG) surgery can be observed in patients with concomitant presence of viable myocardium and absence of dyssynchrony between papillary muscles.[45]

Magnetic Resonance Imaging

Cardiac magnetic resonance imaging (cMRI) is best suited to evaluate LV function and remodeling. It also permits quantification of both the spatial and transmural extent of infarction. In patients with severe ischemic MR, the severity of posterior papillary muscle region scarring correlates with decreased segmental wall motion and MR early after coronary revascularization and annuloplasty.[46] Routinely assessing scar burden may identify patients for whom annuloplasty alone is insufficient to eliminate MR.

Coronary Angiography

The role of coronary angiography is mainly to assess the extent and severity of coronary artery disease and to evaluate the appropriateness of vessels for percutaneous or surgical revascularization.

Management of Patients with Ischemic MR

Myocardial Revascularization

Revascularization does not necessarily reverse ischemic MR. In 136 patients with moderate ischemic MR undergoing coronary bypass surgery, Aklog et al. showed that half the patients had an improvement in MR, but resolution of MR occurred in only 9%, and 40% had residually moderate or severe MR.[16] The effects of revascularization are likely to depend on the presence and extent of viable myocardium.[44,45]

There is a link between the amount of scarring (defined by contrast enhanced MRI) and the severity of MR, and one study showed that improved posterior wall function after thrombolysis was associated with a lower frequency of MR.[15] The role of viable myocardium in ischemic MR is probably important but unproven.

Cardiac Resynchronization Therapy

CRT acutely reduces the severity of ischemic MR, probably through the combined improvement in LV contractile performance and papillary muscle resynchronization.[17,18] Subsequently, reverse remodeling and decreased tethering of the MV apparatus probably contribute as well. After successful CRT implantation, MR improves in most of the patients, remains unchanged in about 25%, and worsens in a relatively small number of patients.

Medical Treatment

The current medical therapy for heart failure includes ACE-inhibitors, diuretics, spironolactone and β(beta)-blockers, and their beneficial effects on symptoms of heart failure in patients with ischemic MR and LV dysfunction may be dramatic. Various combinations of these drugs are commonly used in these patients for two reasons: to reduce the severity of MR and to reverse or delay the LV remodeling process. Use of afterload-reducing agents, such as ACE-inhibitors, has been shown to reduce the RV and to improve forward output by decreasing the pressure gradient between the LV and the LA.[47,48] A similar effect of reduction in MR is obtained with preload reduction through the use of diuretics that decrease ventricular size and further reduce tethering with a consequent decrease in the RV.[49] The use of ACE-inhibitors and β-blockers is an independent predictor of better long-term survival in patients with ischemic MR and LV dysfunction. This could be due to the effects of ACE-inhibitors and β-blockers on progression of LV remodeling and prevention of sudden death.[50,51]

Surgical Approaches

Valve repair and valve replacement, with or without revascularization, are the two available surgical procedures for the treatment of chronic ischemic MR.

Mitral Valve (MV)Repair

The targets of MV repair in ischemic MR include the annulus, the leaflets, the chordae and the LV. The most commonly used annular procedure is undersized mitral annuloplasty using very small symmetric annuloplasty ring.[52,53] The ultimate goal of the annular procedure is to obtain LV reverse remodeling as a consequence of the disappearance of MR and LV volume overload. The preoperative LV dimensions predict the likelihood of reverse remodeling. The chance that reverse remodeling occurs is low if preoperative end-diastolic diameter exceeds 65 mm and/or end-systolic diameter is more than 51 mm.[54] These findings suggest that baseline LV remodeling plays a key role in the likelihood of reverse remodeling and subsequent favorable long-term outcome. Therefore, beyond these cut-off values an additional surgical approach to restore LV dimension or delay the progressive remodeling can be useful. Recurrence of MR is common after ring annuloplasty and occurs in as many as 30% of the patients. Several clinical, surgical, and echocardiographic parameters have been shown to predict postoperative recurrence. They include the use of pericardial rings, continuing LV remodeling progression,[55] preoperative restrictive diastolic filling pattern,[56] a mitral annular diameter exceeding 3.7 cm, a tenting area of more than 1.6 cm²,[57] and a leaflet angle >45°.[40]

Other possible surgical approaches include the edge-to-edge Alfieri technique,[58] the chordal cutting technique,[26] and several other approaches aimed at reshaping the LV and realign papillary muscles to reduce ischemic MR. To date, their usefulness is unproven.

Mitral Valve Replacement

MV replacement, with or without revascularization for ischemic MR, is associated with high, early, and late mortality and low, long-term survival in early studies.[59] Whenever performed with preservation of the entire subvalvular apparatus, it may represent a valid alternative to mitral annuloplasty in some subgroups of patients. In particular, patients with comorbidities, complex regurgitant jets, and/or severe remodeling of mitral apparatus can be treated with a biological prosthesis.[60]

Indications for Mitral Valve Surgery

Although widely used, there is no evidence that mitral annuloplasty alters long-term patient's outcome. At best, it improves symptoms.[61] In the short term, there is evidence that mitral annuloplasty increases operative risk and doubles operative mortality, particularly in the absence of myocardial viability.

Thus, in patients with ischemic MR, the goal of surgical therapy should, probably, not be to improve survival but rather to improve late functional status and late quality of life. Therefore, patients with severe symptomatic ischemic MR should probably be considered for a combined procedure, associating CABG and mitral ring annuloplasty. Indications for surgery are less clear in patients with mild-to-moderate ischemic MR. High-risk perioperative patients with multiple comorbidities and with mild-to-moderate ischemic MR should probably be treated conservatively with revascularization alone, whereas low-risk perioperative patients with few or no co-morbidities and mild-to-moderate ischemic MR can probably undergo a combined procedure.

References

1. Maisel AS, Gilpin EA, Klein L, Le Winter M, Henning H, Collins D. The murmur of papillary muscle dysfunction in acute myocardial infarction; clinical features and prognostic implications. *Am Heart J.* 1986;112:705-711.
2. Barzilai B, Gessler C Jr, Pérez JE, Schaab C, Jaffe AS. Significance of Doppler-detected mitral regurgitation in acute myocardial infarction. *Am J Cardiol.* 1988;61:220-223.
3. Lehmann KG, Francis CK, Dodge HT. Mitral regurgitation in early myocardial infarction: incidence, clinical detection,

and prognostic implications: TIMI Study Group. *Ann Intern Med.* 1992;117:10-17.

4. Loperfido Loperfido F, Biasucci LM, Pennestri F, et al. Pulsed Doppler echocardiographic analysis of mitral regurgitation after myocardial infarction. *Am J Cardiol.* 1986;58:692-697.

5. Tcheng JE, Jackman JD Jr, Nelson CL, et al. Outcome of patients sustaining acute ischemic mitral regurgitation during myocardial infarction. *Ann Intern Med.* 1992;117: 18-24.

6. Hickey MS, Smith LR, Muhlbaier LH, et al. Current prognosis of ischemic mitral regurgitation. Implications for future management. *Circulation.* 1989;798:I51-I59.

7. Grigioni F, Enriquez-Sarano M, Zehr KJ, Bailey KR, Tajik J. Ischemic mitral regurgitation: long-term outcome and prognostic implications with quantitative Doppler assessment. *Circulation.* 2001;103:1759-1764.

8. He S, Fontaine AA, Schwammenthal E, Yoganathan AP, Levine RA. Integrated mechanism for functional mitral regurgitation: leaflet restriction versus coapting force: in vitro studies. *Circulation.* 1997;96:1826-1834.

9. Roberts WC, Cohen LS. Left ventricular papillary muscles. Description of the normal and a survey of conditions causing them to be abnormal. *Circulation.* 1972;46:138-154.

10. Sharma SK, Seckler J, Israel DH, Borrico S, Ambrose JA. Clinical, angiographic and anatomic findings in acute severe ischemic mitral regurgitation. *Am J Cardiol.* 1992;70: 277-280.

11. Hendren WG, Nemec JJ, Lytle BW, et al. Mitral valve repair for ischemic mitral insufficiency. *Ann Thorac Surg.* 1991;52:1246-1251.

12. Rankin JS, Feneley MP, Hickey MS, et al. A clinical comparison of mitral valve repair versus valve replacement in ischemic mitral regurgitation. *J Thorac Cardiovasc Surg.* 1988;95:165-177.

13. Kaul S, Spotnitz WD, Glasheen WP, Touchstone DA. Mechanism of ischemic mitral regurgitation. An experimental evaluation. *Circulation.* 1991;84:2167-2180.

14. Levine RA, Schwammenthal E. Ischemic mitral regurgitation on the threshold of a solution: from paradoxes to unifying concepts. *Circulation.* 2005;112:745-758.

15. Tenenbaum A, Leor J, Motro M, et al. Improved posterobasal segment function after thrombolysis is associated with decreased incidence of significant mitral regurgitation in a first inferior myocardial infarction. *J Am Coll Cardiol.* 1995;25:1558-1563.

16. Aklog L, Filsoufi F, Flores KQ, et al. Does coronary artery bypass grafting alone correct moderate ischemic mitral regurgitation? *Circulation.* 2001;104:I68-I75.

17. Breithardt OA, Sinha AM, Schwammenthal E, et al. Acute effects of cardiac resynchronization therapy on functional mitral regurgitation in advanced systolic heart failure. *J Am Coll Cardiol.* 2003;41:765-770.

18. Kanzaki H, Bazaz R, Schwartzman D, Dohi K, Sade LE, Gorscan J 3rd. A mechanism for immediate reduction in mitral regurgitation after cardiac resynchronization therapy: insights from mechanical activation strain mapping. *J Am Coll Cardiol.* 2004;44:1619-1625.

19. Levine HJ, Gaasch WH. Vasoactive drugs in chronic regurgitant lesions of the mitral and aortic valves. *J Am Coll Cardiol.* 1996;28:1083-1091.

20. Heinle SK, Tice FD, Kisslo J. Effect of dobutamine stress echocardiography on mitral regurgitation. *J Am Coll Cardiol.* 1994;25:122-127.

21. Kizilbash AM, Willett DL, Brickner ME, Heinle SK, Grayburn PA. Effects of afterload reduction on vena contracta width in mitral regurgitation. *J Am Coll Cardiol.* 1998;32:427-431.

22. Godley RW, Wann LS, Rogers EW, Feigenbaum H, Weyman AE. Incomplete mitral leaflet closure in patients with papillary muscle dysfunction. *Circulation.* 1981;63:565-571.

23. Yiu SF, Enriquez-Sarano M, Tribouilloy C, Seward JB, Tajik AJ. Determinants of the degree of functional mitral regurgitation in patients with systolic left ventricular dysfunction. A quantitative clinical study. *Circulation.* 2000;102: 1400-1406.

24. Agricola E, Oppizzi M, Maisano F, et al. Echocardiographic classification of chronic ischemic mitral regurgitation caused by restricted motion according to tethering pattern. *Eur J Echocardiogr.* 2004;5:326-334.

25. Agricola E, Oppizzi M, Pisani M, Meris A, Maisano F, Margonato A. Ischemic mitral regurgitation: mechanisms and echocardiographic classification. *Eur J Echocardiogr.* 2007;9:207-221.

26. Messas E, Guerrero JL, Handschumacher MD, et al. Chordal cutting: a new therapeutic approach for ischemic mitral regurgitation. *Circulation.* 2001;104:1958-1963.

27. Salgo IS, Gorman JH 3rd, Gorman RC, et al. Effect of annular shape on leaflet curvature in reducing mitral leaflet stress. *Circulation.* 2002;106:711-717.

28. Watanabe N, Ogasawara Y, Yamaura Y, et al. Mitral annulus flattens in ischemic mitral regurgitation: geometric differences between inferior and anterior myocardial infarction: a realtime 3-dimensional echocardiographic study. *Circulation.* 2005;112:I1458-I1462.

29. Ahmad RM, Gillinov AM, McCarthy PM, Blackstone EH, et al. Annular geometry and motion in human ischemic mitral regurgitation: novel assessment with three-dimensional echocardiography and computer reconstruction. *Ann Thorac Surg.* 2004;78:2063-2068.

30. De Simone R, Wolf I, Mottl-Link S, et al. A clinical study of annular geometry and dynamics in patients with ischemic mitral regurgitation: new insights into asymmetrical ring annuloplasty. *Eur J Cardiothorac Surg.* 2006;29:355-361.

31. Otsuji Y, Kumanohoso T, Yoshifuku S, et al. Isolated annular dilation does not usually cause important functional mitral regurgitation: comparison between patients with lone atrial fibrillation and those with idiopathic or ischemic cardiomyopathy. *J Am Coll Cardiol.* 2002;39:1651-1656.

32. He S, Lemmon JD Jr, Weston MW, Jensen MO, Levine RA, Yoganathan AP. Mitral valve compensation for annular dilatation: in vitro study into the mechanisms of functional mitral regurgitation with an adjustable annulus model. *J Heart Valve Dis.* 1999;8:294-302.

33. Lapu-Bula R, Robert A, Vancrayenest D, et al. Contribution of exercise-induced mitral regurgitation to exercise stroke volume and exercise capacity in patients with dilated cardiomyopathy. *Circulation.* 2002;106:1342-1348.

34. Lancellotti P, Lebrun F, Pierard LA. Determinants of exercise-induced changes in mitral regurgitation in patients with coronary artery disease and left ventricular dysfunction. *J Am Coll Cardiol.* 2003;42:1921-1928.

35. Zoghbi WA, Enriquez-Sarano M, Foster E, et al. American Society of Echocardiography. Recommendations for evaluation of the severity of native valvular regurgitation with two-dimensional and Doppler echocardiography. *J Am Soc Echocardiogr*. 2003;16:777-802.

36. Matsumura Y, Fukuda S, Tran H, et al. Geometry of the proximal isovelocity surface area in mitral regurgitation by 3-dimensional color Doppler echocardiography: difference between functional mitral regurgitation and prolapse regurgitation. *Am Heart J*. 2008;155:231-238.

37. Matsumura Y, Saracino G, Sugioka K, et al. Determination of regurgitant orifice area with the use of a new three-dimensional flow convergence geometric assumption in functional mitral regurgitation. *J Am Soc Echocardiogr*. 2008;21:1251-1256.

38. Schwammenthal E, Chen C, Benning F, Block M, Breithardt G, Levine RA. Dynamics of mitral regurgitant flow and orifice area. Physiologic application of the proximal flow convergence method: clinical data and experimental testing. *Circulation*. 1994;90:307-322.

39. Buck T, Plicht B, Kahlert P, Schenk IM, Hunold P, Erbel R. Effect of dynamic flow rate and orifice area on mitral regurgitant stroke volume quantification using the proximal isovelocity surface area method. *J Am Coll Cardiol*. 2008;52:767-778.

40. Magne J, Pibarot P, Dagenais F, Hachicha Z, Dumesnil JG, Sénéchal M. Preoperative posterior leaflet angle accurately predicts outcome after restrictive mitral valve annuloplasty for ischemic mitral regurgitation. *Circulation*. 2007;115:782-791.

41. Watanabe N, Ogasawara Y, Yamaura Y, et al. Quantitation of mitral valve tenting in ischemic mitral regurgitation by transthoracic real-time three-dimensional echocardiography. *J Am Coll Cardiol*. 2005;45:763-769.

42. Lancellotti P, Troisfontaines P, Toussaint AC, Pierard LA. Prognostic importance of exercise-induced changes in mitral regurgitation in patients with chronic ischemic left ventricular dysfunction. *Circulation*. 2003;108:1713-1717.

43. Vanoverschelde J-L, Pasquet A, Gerber BL, Melin LA. Principles of myocardial viability. Implications for echocardiography. In: Kisslo J, Nihoyannopoulos P, eds. *Echocardiography*. London: Springer; 2009:351-365.

44. de Waroux JB Le Polain, Pouleur AC, Vancraeynest D, et al. Early hazards of mitral ring annuloplasty in patients with moderate to severe ischemic mitral regurgitation undergoing coronary revascularization: the importance of preoperative myocardial viability. *J Heart Valve Dis*. 2009;18:35-43.

45. Penicka M, Linkova H, Lang O, et al. Predictors of improvement of unrepaired moderate ischemic mitral regurgitation in patients undergoing elective isolated coronary artery bypass graft surgery. *Circulation*. 2009;120:1474-1481.

46. Flynn M, Curtin R, Nowicki ER, et al. Regional wall motion abnormalities and scarring in severe functional ischemic mitral regurgitation: A pilot cardiovascular magnetic resonance imaging study. *J Thorac Cardiovasc Surg*. 2009;137:1063-1070.

47. Stevenson LW, Bellil D, Grover-McKay M, et al. Effects of afterload reduction (diuretics and vasodilators) on left ventricular volume and mitral regurgitation in severe congestive heart failure secondary to ischemic or idiopathic dilated cardiomyopathy. *Am J Cardiol*. 1987;60:654-658.

48. Levine AB, Muller C, Levine TB. Effects of high-dose lisinopril-isosorbide dinitrate on severe mitral regurgitation and heart failure remodeling. *Am J Cardiol*. 1998;82:1299-1301.

49. Bonet S, Agusti A, Arnau JM, et al. Beta-adrenergic blocking agents in heart failure: benefits of vasodilating and non-vasodilating agents according to patients' characteristics: a meta-analysis of clinical trials. *Arch Intern Med*. 2000;160:621-627.

50. Lowes BD, Gill EA, Abraham WT, et al. Effects of carvedilol on left ventricular mass, chamber geometry, and mitral regurgitation in chronic heart failure. *Am J Cardiol*. 1999;83:1201-1205.

51. Capomolla S, Febo O, Gnemmi M, et al. Beta-blockade therapy in chronic heart failure: diastolic function and mitral regurgitation improvement by carvedilol. *Am Heart J*. 2000;139:596-608.

52. Bolling SF, Pagani FD, Deeb GM, Bach DS. Intermediate term outcome of mitral reconstruction in cardiomyopathy. *J Thorac Cardiovasc Surg*. 1998;115:381-386.

53. Bax JJ, Braun J, Somer ST, et al. Restrictive annuloplasty and coronary revascularization in ischemic mitral regurgitation results in reverse left ventricular remodeling. *Circulation*. 2004;110:II103-II108.

54. Braun J, Bax JJ, Versteegh MI, et al. Preoperative left ventricular dimensions predict reverse remodeling following restrictive mitral annuloplasty in ischemic mitral regurgitation. *Eur J Cardiothorac Surg*. 2005;27:847-853.

55. Hung J, Papakostas L, Tahta SA, et al. Mechanism of recurrent ischemic mitral regurgitation after annuloplasty: continued LV remodeling as a moving target. *Circulation*. 2004;110:II85-II90.

56. Ereminiene E, Vaskelyte J, Benetis R, Stoskute N. Ischemic mitral valve repair: predictive significance of restrictive left ventricular diastolic filling. *Echocardiography*. 2005;22:217-224.

57. Kongsaerepong V, Shiota M, Gillinov AM, et al. Echocardiographic predictors of successful versus unsuccessful mitral valve repair in ischemic mitral regurgitation. *Am J Cardiol*. 2006;98:504-508.

58. De Bonis M, Lapenna E, La Canna G, et al. Mitral valve repair for functional mitral regurgitation in end-stage dilated cardiomyopathy: role of the "edge-to-edge" technique. *Circulation*. 2005;112:I402-I408.

59. Akins CW, Hilgenberg AD, Buckley MJ, et al. Mitral valve reconstruction versus replacement for degenerative or ischemic mitral regurgitation. *Ann Thorac Surg*. 1994;58:668-675.

60. Gillinov AM, Wierup PN, Blackstone EH, et al. Is repair preferable to replacement for ischemic mitral regurgitation? *J Thorac Cardiovasc Surg*. 2001;122:1125-1141.

61. Vahanian A, Baumgartner H, Bax J, et al. Guidelines on the management of valvular heart disease: The Task Force on the Management of Valvular Heart Disease of the European Society of Cardiology. *Eur Heart J*. 2007;28:230-268.

Asymptomatic Mitral Valve Regurgitation: Watchful Wait or Early Repair? Review of the Current Evidence

5

Ben Bridgewater and Simon G. Ray

Introduction

Mitral valve(MV) repair for severe mitral regurgitation (MR) secondary to degenerative MV disease is an accepted treatment for patients with symptoms, and for those without symptoms but with decreased left ventricle (LV) systolic function or an increase in left ventricular end systolic dimension. Successive clinical guidelines, over recent years, have suggested that surgery should be offered increasingly early in the disease process. The most recent ACC/AHA guideline suggests that it is reasonable to offer mitral repair to asymptomatic patients with severe MR and normal left ventricular size/function as long as the center is experienced in repair and likelihood of successful repair is high. This chapter will explore the evidence behind these recommendations, and their potential implications.

Severe Mitral Regurgitation

Severe MR due to degenerative disease is a sinister condition that has a high morbidity and mortality if left untreated; patients who have NYHA class III/IV symptoms have a 34% annual mortality in the absence of surgical treatment.[1] The natural history of severe degenerative MR in the absence of surgery is of progressive dilation of the left atrium and LV. Left ventricular ejection fraction is initially maintained due to the high stroke volume, which may mask the onset of underlying contractile dysfunction. Even the slightest drop in ejection fraction (EF) is important. With unchecked regurgitation, patients commonly develop pulmonary hypertension and atrial fibrillation (AF). At some stage, as the disease progresses, symptoms will develop.

Successful surgery is a good treatment for severe MR as it improves both symptoms and life expectancy and, whilst it has never been proven in randomized clinical studies, mitral repair is generally accepted to be a better treatment than mitral replacement for degenerative valvular disease.[2,3] Overall, the outcomes for mitral repair are good, but it has been clearly shown that results are best if surgery is undertaken earlier in the disease; if severe symptoms or left ventricular impairment has developed prior to surgery, survival is significantly worse than it is following "earlier" intervention.[4–7]

Existing Guidelines

Over the last 10 years, there has been an evolution of guidance towards offering earlier and earlier surgery for MR. The 1998 ACC/AHA guidelines recommended surgery for asymptomatic patients with severe MR and AF, pulmonary hypertension, or LV end systolic diameter over 4.5 cm. The most recent ACC/AHA guideline was published in 2006 and was subjected to a targeted update in 2008.[8] This suggests that surgery should be offered to asymptomatic patients when LV systolic dimension size is greater

B. Bridgewater (✉)
Department of Cardiothoracic Surgery, University Hospital of South Manchester, NHS Foundation Trust, Manchester, England
e-mail: ben.bridgewater@uhsm.nhs.uk

R.S. Bonser et al. (eds.), *Mitral Valve Surgery*,
DOI: 10.1007/978-1-84996-426-5_5, © Springer-Verlag London Limited 2011

than 40 mm and also that "MV repair is reasonable in experienced surgical centers for asymptomatic patients with chronic severe MR with preserved LV function (EF greater than 0.60 and end-systolic dimension less than 40 mm) in whom the likelihood of successful repair without residual MR is greater than 90%."[8] This is a class IIa recommendation. The exact wording of this recommendation is important – for surgery to be beneficial at the early stage it is important that repair rather than replacement is performed, it is essential that surgery can be undertaken with minimal morbidity and mortality, and the repair must be effective and leave patients with a high quality long-lasting result with no significant residual regurgitation. The 2007 European guidelines on valvular disease basically reiterate the American document with exception that the threshold for LV end-systolic dimension remained at 45 mm rather than 40 mm.[9] This is an important difference but the European guidelines also state that although there is no data on indexed dimensions, smaller dimensions could be used in smaller patients.

Current State of Valve Repair

There is abundant evidence that mitral repair for severe MR is an underused treatment. The EuroHEART survey reported in 2003 found that 50% of all operations for MR were replacements rather than repair, and 30% of the replacements were thought to be carried out due to lack of local availability of mitral repair expertise.[10] There have been similar findings reported in the United States, where only 30% of operations for MR were repairs, and the majority of these were annuloplasty alone. The majority of mitral repair operations still seem to be carried out at a late stage in the disease with 48% of patients in the EuroHEART survey being in NYHA class III or IV. A recent analysis of the Society for Cardiothoracic Surgery (SCTS) in Great Britain and Ireland national database of over 5,000 mitral repairs suggested over 40% were in NYHA class III or IV and only 16% of patients were in NYHA class I with good LV function.[11] It is not known how many of these patients had significant dilatation of the LV as the indication for surgery.

What Is the Outcome of Patients with Asymptomatic Severe Mitral Regurgitation?

A substantial amount of the evidence base on which current mitral repair practice is founded has come from researchers at the Mayo Clinic. They have held a view for some time that very early surgery for MR is beneficial. As long ago as 1997, Ling et al. described the outcomes of 221 patients undergoing mitral repair surgery for isolated degenerative severe MR.[6] Sixty-three of these underwent "early" surgery, within a month of diagnosis, with the remainder undergoing "conservative" management and 80 of this group subsequently underwent surgery. The early surgery group were younger and more likely to be symptomatic or in AF. The early surgery group had a better survival and a better postoperative cardiovascular physiology than the conservative group and early surgery came out as an independent predictor of better outcome and decreased cardiovascular mortality in multi-variate analysis.

To subject asymptomatic patients to cardiac surgery as an essentially "prophylactic" measure is a major undertaking. Two more studies in recent years have aimed to address the outcomes for these patients in the absence of surgery, and have come up with somewhat conflicting findings. A recent publication, again from the Mayo Clinic, evaluated 456 patients with asymptomatic organic MR with quantitative echo and evaluated their outcomes.[12] Outcomes at 5 years were worse than expected for those who had moderate or severe regurgitation. About 50% of the patients underwent surgery with a mean time from diagnosis to operation of 15 months, with an overall 30-day mortality of 1% with 91% receiving a repair procedure. They found that increasing age, diabetes, and increasing effective regurgitant orifice area (EROA) were independent predictors of a poor outcome and that patients with EROA >40 mm^2 had a 5-year survival that was lower than expected. Quantitative grading of MR was a powerful predictor of outcome and they recommend that patients with an EROA >40 mm^2 should promptly be considered for surgery.

It is not straightforward to extrapolate the findings from this study more widely for two reasons; those of imaging and the quality of mitral repair services. Most echo labs do not routinely quantify MR in the way described in this study and rely more on a semi-quantitative approach using a combination of factors as described below, but it is probably not an accurate measurement of EROA, which is important in determining prognosis; however, very severe MR is identified in a reliable way. The quality of mitral repair at the Mayo Clinic is likely to be of the very highest standard, with repair being performed routinely in large volumes by surgeons with significant subspecialist expertise. This is not always the case in other institutions.

An alternative approach for these asymptomatic patients is to pursue a "watchful waiting" policy and to intervene as soon as symptoms or features of cardiac dysfunction develop. This has been reported to be a safe strategy by Rosenhek et al.[13] They looked at 138 patients with severe asymptomatic MR according to a methodological, integrated approach to the semiquantitative assessment of MR as described by the American Society of Echo. Fifty-eight of these patients had flail mitral leaflets. They enrolled these patients into a careful follow-up protocol and intervened according to existing published guidelines at that time of symptoms, LV dysfunction, new onset AF or pulmonary hypertension or dilation of the LV to a systolic diameter of greater than 4.5 cm. Thirty-eight patients (less than third) underwent surgery over the study period (with no intra-operative deaths); the overall 8-year survival was 91%.

To reiterate, if an early intervention strategy is to be considered, it is imperative that surgery is of the highest quality, operative mortality and morbidity is negligible, patients are not subjected to valve replacements with their inherent problems, and incidence of residual regurgitation is low. Even if an early surgery strategy is followed, it is quite possible that some patients will be subjected to the risks and inconvenience of surgery, in whom it might never have become necessary had a watchful waiting policy been followed. Similarly, the watchful waiting strategy is safe only if processes for follow-up are absolutely robust. If patients become lost to follow-up or develop significant undetected symptoms or LV abnormalities during follow-up, these patients will not derive the optimal benefit from subsequent mitral surgery.

The chances of a successful and long-lasting repair also depend on the exact nature of the valvular abnormality. Isolated prolapse of the posterior leaflet is the commonest abnormality and the easiest to repair and, in general, there will be a good long-lasting outcome following surgery, but there is a small risk (which will depend on the operator) of intra-operative replacement rather than repair, and a risk of re-operation of about 0.5% per year, which will again be operator dependent. Anterior leaflet disease will have higher intra-operative and postoperative risk of failure.[14] The decision about timing of surgery for asymptomatic patients should, therefore, be made cognizant of the exact leaflet pathology against the expertise and experience of available surgical mitral repair surgery.

Echocardiographic Assessment

Echocardiography is essential to the assessment of MR and particularly so in guiding surgical decision making in asymptomatic patients. It should answer a number of specific questions:

- What is the severity of the regurgitation?
- What is the etiology and mechanism of the regurgitation?
- What is the LV function?
- What other abnormalities are present?

Severity of Mitral Regurgitation

Wherever possible, quantitative estimation of the severity of MR should be performed.[15] Of the available quantitative methods, the most widely used is utilizing proximal isovelocity surface area (PISA). This method is technically demanding, requires practice, and must be used routinely if it is to be clinically useful. Quantitative methods can be used to calculate both RV and EROA. EROA is more closely associated with outcome and should be the standard measure used. An EROA of 40 mm^2 or greater is consistent with severe MR.[14] However, no single parameter should be used alone and other measures of regurgitation should be used to provide confirmatory evidence of severity.[15] Basic eyeballing methods such as the area of the color flow jet or the presence of reversed systolic flow in the pulmonary veins are inadequate unless performed as part of a systematic assessment. Only those patients with a secure diagnosis of severe regurgitation should be considered for surgery, and this is applicable to all patients, but particularly pertinent to the asymptomatic patients where the risk-benefit equation is more finely balanced.

Etiology and Mechanism

If mitral valve repair is to be undertaken in asymptomatic patients then the echocardiographic assessment must be made in a systematic fashion and the pathology and likely repair precisely described. It is possible, with experience, to identify the etiology and mechanism of the regurgitation in the majority of cases using standardized views on 2D transthoracic echocardiography. Routine preoperative transoesophageal echocardiography (TOE) is not necessary in an established mitral repair service, but where there is doubt about the cause of the MR, then TOE or three-dimensional echocardiography (TTE or TOE) can provide additional information.[16,17]

As described above, what is repairable by one surgeon is not necessarily repairable by another and cases must be assessed and discussed on an individual basis in the light of local experience.

Left Ventricular Function

The large stroke volume associated with severe MR may mask the development of left ventricular contractile dysfunction. As in the assessment of regurgitant severity, simple "eyeballing" is inadequate and EF should be calculated in every patient. Any reduction in EF below 60% should be regarded as abnormal and a potential indication for early surgery. Its marked load dependency makes EF a far-from ideal method to assess contractile function in chronic severe MR but it is a relatively simple measurement to make and is known to predict outcome. Ventricular dysfunction secondary to volume overload is global and any focal wall motion abnormality should prompt a search for an ischemic cause.

There is emerging evidence that newer techniques might be able to detect subclinical LV dysfunction. Tissue Doppler strain rate has been shown to be higher in patients with intact contractile reserve but has inherent problems with signal-to-noise ratio.[18] Speckle tracking methods may also be useful, but they are as yet clinically unproven.[19]

Other Abnormalities

The echocardiographic assessment should include the potential secondary consequences of MR, particularly pulmonary hypertension. Asymptomatic patients with good left ventricular function but elevated pulmonary pressures (>50 mmHg) have an established indication for surgery.[8] Where pulmonary pressures are borderline, exercise echo is worthwhile as an exercise. PA systolic pressure of >60 mmHg is also an indication for consideration of operation.

The Place of Exercise Testing and Exercise Echocardiography

The onset of symptoms in patients with MR may be insidious, especially in older, less active subjects. Functional capacity on cardiopulmonary exercise testing is unexpectedly abnormal in 20–25% of asymptomatic patients with severe MR and a reduction in VO2 max below 84% of predicted is associated with an adverse outcome.[20] If there is any doubt about symptom status in patients with severe MR, then exercise testing should be performed, ideally cardiopulmonary testing, and an otherwise unexplained reduction in functional capacity should prompt serious consideration of early surgery.[8]

Exercise echocardiography may also be useful. Failure of contractile reserve defined as an increase in LV EF of <4% on exercise is associated with a worse outcome and could prompt earlier operation.[21] As discussed above, pulmonary pressures should also be estimated during exercise as a rise in PA pressure to >60 mmHg is a class IIa indication for surgery according to the AHA/ACC guidelines.

Frequency of Review

If a decision is made to defer surgery, then asymptomatic patients under review should be seen every 6 months with detailed echocardiography. Casual outpatient review is inadequate.

Studies on Improving Mitral Services

The progression of guidelines for treatment of patients with asymptomatic MR over the last 10 years has been towards earlier surgery but, as described above, there do seem to be significant variations in the availability of high quality mitral repair services.

In an analysis of the STS database of over of 13,614 patients in the United States who had either repair or replacement for MR with an overall in-hospital mortality of 2.1%, investigators found that larger volume centers were likely to have a better chance of repairing (rather than replacing) the valve, were more likely to undertake surgery in asymptomatic patients, and showed lower risk-adjusted mortality.[22] It is possible to marshal an argument that all patients undergoing essentially "prophylactic" mitral repair surgery should be referred to these largest centers. Various authors have suggested that it is possible to improve the quality of mitral surgery by reconfiguring services, and concentrating surgical expertise in fewer hands, with dedicated subspecialist teams. Data from a large surgical practice in the United States underline the importance of appropriate referral by cardiologists. Of 18 surgeons, two performed more than 20 mitral valve repairs per year whilst the remaining 16 surgeons each performed less than 20. This second group performed 49% of all repairs undertaken by the service but had a repair rate of only 18%. The two higher volume surgeons performed 51% of repairs with a repair rate of 51%.[23] A patient referred to a higher volume surgeon had an approximately threefold greater chance of a repair. There are also data to confirm that a team approach works well. In a Californian center, concentration of the management of all mitral prolapse patients in the hands of a single cardiologist and a single surgeon and the introduction of a dedicated intraoperative TOE

service resulted in a dramatic increase in repair rates and a corresponding reduction in the number of valve replacements.[24]

A multi-disciplinary publication from the United Kingdom has defined "best practice" standard for mitral valve repair including suggested volume thresholds and outcomes targets.[25] The latest ACC/AHA guidance has tried to drive this process by suggesting that "cardiologists are strongly advised to refer patients for valve repair to experienced centers" and has suggested that surgery for asymptomatic patients should only be considered in experienced surgical centers, in patients where the likelihood of successful repair without residual regurgitation is better than 90%.

In our view, there is an onus on both cardiologists and cardiac surgeons to ensure that patients with asymptomatic severe MR and preserved LV function are optimally treated. Cardiologists lacking a clear understanding of the repairability of a mitral valve are more likely to accept their patient receiving a replacement. It should no longer be acceptable for a cardiologist to refer for "valve surgery" without informed consideration of the best option for an individual patient and cardiologists unsure of the repairability of a particular valve should be able to refer to a colleague with a specialist interest. Similarly, cardiac surgeons acting in the best interests of their patients must be prepared to refer patients on to colleagues if they are not confident of performing a specific repair.

IS There a Need for a Randomized Study?

The data on patients undergoing medical and surgical therapy with severe MR are based entirely on observational studies, with all the inherent potentials for bias, and is heavily dependent on reports from highly experienced, expert centers. Randomized studies have the ability to give a clear answer about whether asymptomatic patients with normal left ventricular size and function will benefit from early surgery. Looking at the available data, a significant cardiac event rate (death for cardiac causes, heart failure or new AF) as high as 33% has been reported by 5 years after diagnosis in untreated patients, and such a study to detect a significant reduction in a combined end point would potentially be possible with a large national/international multicenter study.

References

1. Ling LH, Enriquez-Sarano M, Seward JB, et al. Clinical outcome of mitral regurgitation due to flail leaflet. *N Engl J Med*. 1996;335:1417-1423.
2. Enriquez-Sarano M, Schaff HV, Orszulak TA, et al. Valve repair improves the outcome of surgery for mitral regurgitation. A multivariate analysis. *Circulation*. 1995;91:1022-1028.
3. Lee EM, Shapiro LM, Wells FC. Superiority of mitral valve repair in surgery for degenerative mitral regurgitation. *Eur Heart J*. 1997;18:655-663.
4. Ling LH, Enriquez-Sarano M, Seward JB, et al. Clinical outcome of mitral regurgitation due to flail leaflet. *N Engl J Med*. 1996;335:1417-1423.
5. Enriquez-Sarano M, Tajik AJ, Schaff HV, Orszulak TA, Bailey KR, Frye RL. Echocardiographic prediction of survival after surgical correction of organic mitral regurgitation. *Circulation*. 1994;90(2):830-837.
6. Ling LH, Enriquez-Sarano M, Seward JB, et al. Early surgery in patients with mitral regurgitation due to flail leaflets: a long-term outcome study. *Circulation*. 1997; 96(6):1819-1825.
7. Tribouilloy CM, Enriquez-Sarano M, Schaff HV, et al. Impact of preoperative symptoms on survival after surgical correction of organic mitral regurgitation: rationale for optimizing surgical indications. *Circulation*. 1999;99(3):400-5.
8. Bonow RO, Carabello BA, Chatterjee K, et al. ACC/AHA 2006 Guidelines for the management of patients with valvular heart disease. *J Am Coll Cardiol*. 2006;48(3):e1.
9. Monin JL, Dehant P, Roiron C, et al. Guidelines on the management of valvular heart disease. *Eur Heart J*. 2007; 28:230-268.
10. Lung B, Baron G, Butchart EG, et al. A prospective survey of patients with valvular heart disease in Europe: The Euro Heart Survey on Valvular Heart Disease. *Eur Heart J*. 2003; 24:1231-1243.
11. Bridgewater B, Kinsman R, Walton P, Keogh B. *Demonstrating quality: the sixth National Adult Cardiac Surgical Database report*. Henley-on-Thames, Oxfordshire: Dendrite Clinical Sytems; 2009.
12. Enriquez-Sarano M, Avierinos JF, Messika-Zeitoun D, et al. Quantitative determinants of the outcome of asymptomatic mitral regurgitation. *N Engl J Med*. 2005;352:875-883.
13. Rosenhek R, Rader F, Klaar U, et al. Outcome of watchful waiting in asymptomatic severe mitral regurgitation. *Circulation*. 2006;113(18):2238-44.
14. Suri RM, Schaff HV, Dearani JA, et al. Survival advantage and improved durability of mitral repair for leaflet prolapse subsets in the current era. *Ann Thorac Surg*. 2006;82(3): 819-826.
15. Zoghbi WA, Enriquez-Sarano M, Foster E, et al. Recommendations for evaluation of the severity of native valvular regurgitation with two dimensional and Doppler echocardiography. *J Am Soc Echocardiogr*. 2003;16:777-802.
16. Pepi M, Tamborini G, Maltagliati A, et al. Head to head comparison of two and three dimensional TTE and TOE in the localisation of mitral valve prolapse. *JACC*. 2006;48: 2524-2530.
17. McNab A, Jenkins NP, Ewington I, et al. A method for the morphological analysis of the regurgitant mitral valve using three-dimensional echocardiography. *Heart*. 2004;90: 771-776.
18. Lee R, Hanekom L, Marwick TH, Wahi S. Prediction of sub clinical LV dysfunction with strain rate imaging in patients with asymptomatic severe mitral regurgitation. *Am J Cardiol*. 2004;94:1333-1340.
19. Borg AN, Harrison AN, Argyle RAM, Ray SG. Left ventricular torsion in primary chronic mitral regurgitation. *Heart*. 2008;94(5):597-603.
20. Messika-Zeitoun D, Johnson BD, Nkomo V, et al. Cardiopulmonary exercise testing determination of functional capacity in mitral regurgitation: physiologic and outcome determinants. *JACC*. 2006;47:2521-2527.
21. Lee R, Haluska B, Deung DY, Case C, Mundy J, Marwick TH. Functional and prognostic implications of left ventricular contractile reserve in patients with asymptomatic severe mitral regurgitation. *Heart*. 2005;91:1407-1421.
22. Gammie JS, O'Brien SM, Griffith BP, Ferguson TB, Peterson ED. Influence of hospital procedural volume on care process and mortality for patients undergoing elective surgery for mitral regurgitation. *Circulation*. 2007;115(7):881-887. Epub 2007 Feb 5.
23. Northrup WF III. Mitral valve repair: we must do a better job. *Curr Cardiol Rep*. 2005;7:94-100.
24. Matsunaga A, Shah PM, Raney AA Jr. Impact of intraoperative echocardiography/surgery team on successful mitral valve repair: a community hospital experience. *J Heart Valve Dis*. 2005;14(3):325-330.
25. Bridgewater B, Hooper TL, Munsch C, et al. Mitral repair best practice: proposed standards. *Heart*. 2006;92(7): 939-944.

Introduction

The atrio-ventricular valves (tricuspid and mitral) are characterized by their connections to their respective ventricles by tendinous chords that arise from muscular projections from within the ventricular walls, the papillary muscles. Within the left ventricle, there are two principal papillary muscles whose names are derived from their anatomical positions within the left ventricle. They are the antero-lateral and postero-medial papillary muscles. These muscle projections are composed of muscle fibers that descend from the base of the ventricle and then turn inward and upward to extend as vertical fibers, which form the papillary muscles.[1] Each papillary muscle gives rise to tendinous chords that insert into both aortic and mural leaflets, which are fan-shaped at the commissures. They, with the mitral valve leaflets, form a ventricular inflow tract for the blood leaving the left atrium (Fig. 6.1). There are three tiers of tendinous chords extending from the papillary muscles and are referred to as the primary, secondary, and tertiary chords. The primary chords insert into the leading edge of the leaflets, guiding them into early apposition; the secondary chords are responsible for load transference into the body of the leaflets; the tertiary chords are found in relation to the mural leaflet. They usually arise from the ventricular wall or toward the base of the papillary muscles and insert into the base of the leaflet at its origin from the atrio-ventricular junction.[2] They are loaded throughout the cardiac cycle, acting rather like "tie-rods" in an engineering sense.

This structural arrangement results in a functional continuity, which is referred to as the atrio-ventricular loop. The closed and fully loaded leaflets resist the hydrostatic forces of the compressed blood and the chords relay the engendered forces between the leaflets and the ventricular wall via the contracted papillary muscles. This force field also acts as an important platform for the structural integrity of the tensioned ventricular muscle mass. Excision of the leaflets and chords in the process of mitral valve replacement disrupts this relationship and as a result the ventricular muscle will lose a major part of its structural integrity.

During the initial phase of mitral valve surgery, the importance of this relationship was not appreciated and complete excision of the valve apparatus (leaflets,

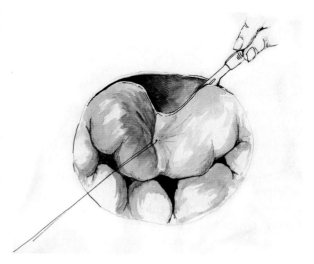

Fig. 6.1 A suture placed through the body of the aortic leaflet retracted toward the surgeon enables very accurate incision and detachment of the leaflet from the atrio-ventricular junction. The whole of the leaflet is then detached and separated from the mural leaflet

F.C. Wells
Department of Cardiac Surgery, Papworth Hospital,
Cambridge, Cambridgeshire, UK
e-mail: francis.wells@papworth.nhs.uk

R.S. Bonser et al. (eds.), *Mitral Valve Surgery*,
DOI: 10.1007/978-1-84996-426-5_6, © Springer-Verlag London Limited 2011

chords, and tips of the papillary muscles) was the norm in replacement surgery. It was only when the results of mitral valve replacement were examined that the impact on ventricular function became clear. It was Lillehei[3] in 1964 who first reported the worrying results of mitral valve replacement where all of the native valve and its ventricular components had been removed. Despite satisfactorily functioning prosthetic valves, approximately 50% of patients were dying from heart failure within 5 years. Postmortem examination of the hearts revealed a globular remodeling of the ventricular cavity. Lillehei recommended that the subvalvar apparatus be preserved at least in part during the procedure of mitral valve replacement surgery in an attempt to preserve normal ventricular integrity.[3]

While the precise activity and timing of the papillary muscle contraction and relaxation throughout the cardiac cycle remains conjectural, it is clear that the disruption of this atrio-ventricular structural loop permanently interrupts the sharing of the forces developed during contraction and relaxation of the ventricular muscle. It has been argued that the normal geometric form of the ventricle tends toward that of a complex cone, that is, a cone with an inherent twist, which is important in the early phase of systole. This natural form engenders a situation where the emptying of the ventricle mimics the wringing out of a towel. This kind of explanation is the answer to the question of how a muscle mass in which none of the constituent muscle fibers can shorten to more than 15% of its length can produce ventricular chamber emptying of up to 70% of its volume. This conundrum has been discussed by Ingels.[4]

The structural arrangement of the myocardium has been discussed at length over many years, but a true consensus on the actual mechanism of chamber contraction leading to ejection has yet to be arrived at. The easiest mechanistic explanation for this would be a helical arrangement of the heart muscle fiber orientation. This was first proposed and demonstrated by R. Lower in 1669.[5] Recently, the hypothesis of a "spiral" myocardial band, first raised by Lower centuries ago, has been developed by Torrent-Guasp[6] and championed by Buckberg.[7] They suggest that the myocardial fibers are arranged in a helical fashion in such a way that the heart can be unfurled. However, the veracity of this work has been challenged by Anderson et al who contradict this gross morphological arrangement as false. They rather

place the emphasis on the myocyte arrangement at a microscopic level to produce this functional outcome,[8] suggesting that the method used to demonstrate the furled helix produces an artificial construct through the denaturation of the natural bonds within the myocardium allowing separation in any desired plane. Pettigrew[9] demonstrated the changing fiber orientation of myocyte aggregation at different depths within the myocardium and Brachet at the beginning of the nineteenth century suggested dual components to the myocardium with one group of cells orientated for systolic contraction and another for diastolic movement.[10] Physiological observation suggests that toward the end of diastole, particularly as a result of the atrial "kick" of atrial contraction, the filling of the ventricle is unfurled far beyond its resting state gaining elastic energy from the non-myocyte structural components of the myocardium. At the end of diastole, therefore, this elastic energy injected into the unwound ventricle as a result of this stretching and untwisting begins the recoil of the ventricular mass, which accelerates as active muscular contraction develops. Whatever the mechanism turns out to be when fully understood, repeated studies continue to confirm that the atrio-ventricular loop is an important factor in the transmission of these forces and the maintenance of the normal geometry of the ventricle.[11]

After this relationship has been disrupted by disconnecting the papillary muscles from the base of the heart, the ventricle gradually takes a more globular form and becomes progressively less efficient.[12] The end result is of a significantly earlier mortality through heart failure. Preservation of the subvalve connections when a prosthetic valve is inserted appears to preserve ventricular function.[13,14] Although definitive physiological data is lacking, this detrimental effect seems to be measurable immediately after surgery.[15] Indeed, the detrimental effect is amplified with the passage of time. In our own study comparing mitral valve repair with replacement with subvalve preservation and complete excision, there was only a 63.5± % at 7 years postoperatively for the replacement group without preservation of any subvalve apparatus.[16] This compared badly with both mitral valve repair group and the replacement with subvalve preservation group. Multivariate analysis confirmed independent beneficial effects of repair on 30-day mortality (odds ratio, 0.27, $P < .05$) and of repair and MVR/SVP on overall mortality (hazard ratios, 0.43, *P* <.001 and 0.40, *P* <.05, respectively) and complication-related death (hazard ratios, 0.38, *P* <.001 and 0.35, *P* <.05). Myocardial failure caused 66 of the 107 deaths in this group. In a study using cost as a surrogate for speed and ease of recovery, we were able to show that both mitral valve repair and mitral valve insertion with partial or complete subvalve preservation were superior to mitral valve replacement without any subvalve preservation.[17]

The papillary muscles are only found in the inlet portion of the left ventricle and there is a large portion of the chamber that is not related to the papillary muscles. It is an interesting question, therefore, why this particular anatomical arrangement is so important for normal ventricular function. It is possible that this continuous loop relationship is important for this posterior part of the left ventricle as it is the part that is bounded by the free, and therefore, unsupported portion of the wall of the ventricle unlike the more anterior part, the ventricular outflow channel, which is bounded by the septum and the right ventricle in front of that.

While many surgeons now preserve part of, or the entire, mural leaflet, the anterior leaflet frequently continues to be removed along with its chords. It is argued that the preservation of the mural leaflet attachments alone is sufficient. Interestingly, at least one study has shown that the aortic leaflet chordae may make a greater contribution to ventricular function than those of the mural leaflet and the effect of preserving both leaflet connections is additive.[18]

A dread complication of mitral valve surgery is dehiscence of the posterior wall of the left ventricle. This most commonly occurs in the setting of rheumatic mitral stenosis when the whole valve is excised. Thickened and fused mural leaflet chords may also be used in part on the ventricular wall. If the endocardium is inadvertently breached in the excision of this leaflet, the underlying muscle separates and blood under pressure insinuates itself into the ventricular wall causing its disruption. Preservation of the mural leaflet and resisting the temptation to oversize the chosen prosthesis will minimize the risk of this happening.[19]

For all these reasons, surgeons should strive to retain *all* the principal chordal connections when implanting a prosthetic valve. With this goal in mind, there are a variety of strategies that may be adopted to implant the numerous different devices safely and without the interference in valve function by the retained subvalve apparatus.

Surgical Strategies for Preservation of the Atrio-Ventricular Loop During Insertion of a Mitral Prosthesis

The mechanics of the type of valve that is to be implanted is an important consideration when deciding the approach that is to be used in retaining the chordal attachments. When mechanical valves are used, part of the retained subvalve apparatus may insinuate itself between valve leaflets and the valve housing, resulting in obstruction to full and easy opening and closing. Therefore, when using this type of valve, great care must be taken to ensure that there are no excessive projections of leaflet tissue beneath the valve housing. When biological prosthetic valves are used, the retained valve apparatus is shielded by the leaflets and therefore cannot interfere with prosthetic leaflet systolic coaptation. However, it is important to note that tissue valves are not immune from potential problems when the natural valve is preserved. If the retained tissue is excessively bulky, it can prevent full prosthetic leaflet opening. Also, if the whole of the aortic leaflet of the mitral valve is kept and a tissue valve is simply inserted within its orifice, it is possible for the central body of the aortic leaflet to prolapse into the aortic outflow tract in systole and produce left ventricular outflow obstruction, a form of SAM (systolic anterior motion of the aortic leaflet into the outflow tract, more commonly associated with mitral valve repair[20]). Therefore, the amount of tissue that may be retained for the two principal valve types is different and, indeed, should be tailored to accommodate the differing morbid anatomy between valves. Leaflet and chordal preservation during valve insertion in the presence of a Barlow[21] type of myxomatous degeneration where there is voluminous excess leaflet tissue will need to be different than for a typically rheumatic valve, where the tissues are thickened, contracted, and the papillary muscles often fused to the underside of the leaflets and to each other.

Surgical Techniques

Once the decision to insert a prosthetic valve has been taken, proceed as follows. In the presence of an irreparable degenerative valve or a rheumatic valve with relatively pliable leaflets and chords and papillary muscles that are not excessively thickened, retracted, and shortened, the technique that follows can be used.

First, place a stitch through the center of the aortic leaflet to act as a retractor. Pull the leaflet toward yourself and incise the leaflet approximately 1–2 mm away from the atrial reflection. Using scissors or a knife, continue the incision in both directions toward the commissures (Fig. 6.1). When the whole leaflet is freed from the annulus, cut through the center of the aortic leaflet to its coaptation margin (Fig. 6.2a). This separates the leaflet into two approximately triangular portions. The excess leaflet tissue at the apices of these triangles may then be resected, leaving enough tissue to easily support the sutures (Fig. 6.2b). Using the surgeon's preferred suture material, sutures are placed from the atrial surface of the prepared leaflet segment and then into the annulus of the valve from the ventricular side fixing the leaflet margin with all of its attached chords to the underside of the annulus (Fig. 6.3). These same sutures are used to pass through the sewing ring of the prosthetic valve to secure the valve in place.

1. There is usually a gap of 1–2 cm between the two leaflet segments at the top dead center of the valve annulus from the surgeon's perspective. An adequate number of sutures are used to fill this interval for fixation of the prosthetic valve. I prefer pledgeted sutures[1] for this situation to spread the load more evenly across the fixed tissue.

2. The approach to the mural leaflet will depend on the amount and thickness of the tissue available. If the leaflet is narrow and not very thickened or calcified, it may be left in place and gathered up beneath the annulus with the sutures (Fig. 6.4). If the leaflet is very tall, it can be detached from the atrio-ventricular junction and the excess tissue excised. I often find that simply detaching the leaflet, placing the suture through the tissue, and then passing the suture through the ventricular side of the annulus will pull the excess tissue out of the orifice of the valve. Usually, there is a centimeter or two between the insertions of the chords from each papillary muscle head that can be

---

[1]There are a number of different ready prepared proprietary sutures available for this work. Some are braided for extra strength and bear an external wax coating to allow easy passage of the suture through the tissues.

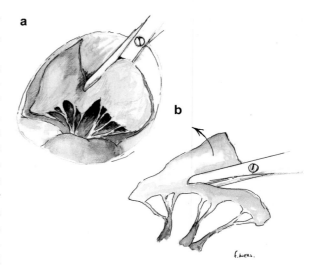

Fig. 6.2 (**a**) The aortic leaflet is then divided in the middle giving two segments of leaflet each with its own chords attached, one segment for each of the principal papillary muscles. (**b**) The triangular segments of excess leaflet tissue are then cut away leaving a sound margin of leaflet tissue attached to the chords through which the valve sutures may be passed

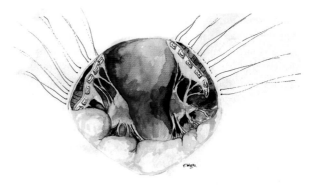

Fig. 6.3 The sutures through each segment of the mural leaflet are then passed through the atrio-ventricular junction, thereby restoring the atrio-ventricular loop

excised, as there are no chords attached to this segment; removing unnecessary tissue reduces the chance of prosthetic leaflet obstruction.

3. The sutures that are now securing the preserved subvalve connections are then passed through the appropriately sized prosthetic valve. It is important not to oversize the chosen valve. It should sit snugly within the orifice. Oversizing is another potential cause of mural ventricular rupture. When the valve is in place, ensure that the leaflets can open and close easily and fully and without obstruction. Small

Fig. 6.4 The mural leaflet may be excised from the atrio-ventricular junction if the leaflet is large. The excessive tissue is then excised and reattached using the valve sutures drawing the retained leaflet margin with attached chords underneath the atrio-ventricular junction. Alternatively, the leaflet tissue may be folded upon itself and gathered up in the stitch, which is then passed in the same way through the atrio-ventricular junction

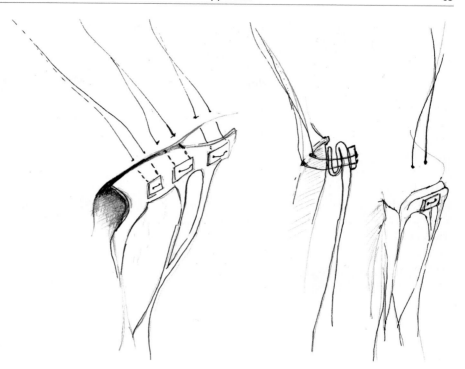

amounts of intrusive excess tissue may be shaved away through the valve, but this is better avoided by trimming the retained tissue to the minimum required for structural integrity. It is not necessary to preserve every single chordal element. Simply select the structurally most important elements and retain the portion of leaflet that they are inserted into.

Valves will be encountered that cannot be managed in this way. If the leaflets and the chords are so thickened and retracted that the leaflets fuse with the papillary muscles, it is often necessary to excise all of the valve and the chords to free the papillary muscles and to create an adequate orifice for the prosthetic valve. All is not lost in these circumstances. New chordal attachments can be created by placing Gore-Tex© sutures between the papillary muscle heads and the valve annulus. These can be taken from each papillary muscle head, which is then reattached to the annulus with pairs of sutures. For this maneuver, I use sutures with small synthetic or pericardial pledgets to evenly distribute the load on the muscular portion of the papillary muscles. This simple technique can be used for part or all of the subvalve apparatus. It can also be used in repeat surgery in patients in whom the whole of the subvalve apparatus has been removed at a previous procedure. It is usually possible to find remnants of the

papillary muscle projections, although it is very salutary to see how much they have been effaced in the negative remodeling of the ventricular wall.

Annular Calcification

Occasionally, significant calcification of the annulus of the mitral valve will be encountered such that there is nowhere to safely place the sutures for the prosthetic valve. The calcification often extends well down into the mural leaflet and onto the chords and papillary muscle, which may become a solid sheet of fibro-calcified tissue. Indeed, in some patients, the calcification may completely encircle the orifice of the valve. The first sign may be seen on a plain chest radiograph. It is important to know the extent of this prior to surgery. Modern cardiac computerized tomogram scans will reveal the extent of the problem in considerable detail, allowing adequate assessment of the problem and a surgical plan that is likely to succeed (Fig. 6.5). There are strategies to deal with this however, which still allow subvalve preservation.

Very occasionally in a particularly elderly patient, especially if significant comorbidities exist, this problem may be so severe as to make surgery unsafe.

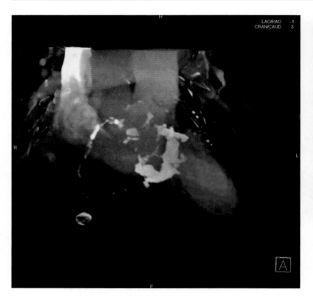

Fig. 6.5 Cardiac CT scan image of peri-annular calcification

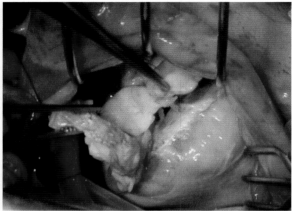

Fig. 6.6 Intra-operative photograph of a large band of calcium being excised from the atrio-ventricular junction after the mural leaflet has been detached

If the calcification is localized, then it may be quite simply excised, taking care not to cut into the ventricular muscle. This can usually be achieved by cutting just onto the edge of the calcified portion and paring away the leaflet and ventricular tissue and lifting out the calcified portion. If the denuded area is small, it may be closed with direct sutures. If it is of a significant size (>1–1.5 cm), then it is best to patch it with a piece of pericardium (either autologous or xenograft pericardium). It is sewn into place using a continuous polypropylene suture of four "0" gauge. The techniques for reattachment of the chordal leaflet remnants, as described above, can then be utilized. Pledgeted sutures with the chords already attached are placed through the pericardial patch and then through the prosthetic valve such that the pericardial patch is sandwiched between valve and chordal leaflet.

If the calcification is extensive, then the calcified area can be excised *en bloc* after any pliable leaflet tissue has been cut away, preserving the chordal attachments (Fig. 6.6). This is best done with a knife, cutting just onto the calcified part at the endocardial reflection rather than directly into the muscle (Fig. 6.7). It is important to proceed cautiously as this is done. When complete, a pericardial patch can be sewn to the edges of the defect. There is usually a tide of fibrous tissue in front of the calcified area, which should be kept as this is very strong to sew to. The pericardial patch should be quite generous in size and the surgeon should not

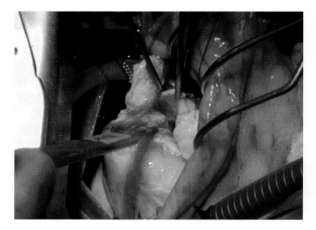

Fig. 6.7 The final stages of excision of the calcified tissue from the atrio-ventricular groove. Note the margin of white fibrous tissue at the ventricular margin

attempt to re-approximate the ventricular muscle to the atrial tissue, as this will result in unnecessary stress on the tissues with the risk of dehiscence (Fig. 6.8). Once the patch is in place, the detached leaflet with the chords still attached can be sewn back to the new annulus using the valve sutures as previously described. The valve can then be inserted. It is important not to oversize the chosen valve so as not to place undue stress on the reconstructed annulus. The midterm results of such an approach have been described by David and colleagues.[22]

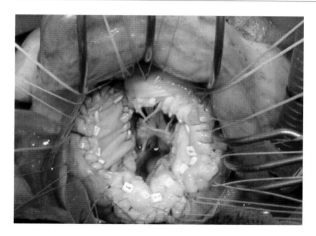

Fig. 6.8 A generous pericardial patch has been sewn into place to re-unite the atrial wall with the ventricular inflow and the sutures to hold the valve in place with partial subvalve preservation are being sited prior to attachment to the sewing ring of the new valve

Other techniques have been described to allow valve insertion in this setting. They include the creation of a pericardial baffle within the left atrium into which the valve is sewn and the inversion of part of the left atrial wall from where sutures are passed to the free edge of the calcified leaflet if there is room and then through the valve.[23] I have not found it necessary to recourse to these techniques thus far.

References

1. Armour JA, Randall WC. Structural basis for cardiac function. *Am J Physiol.* 1970;218:1517.
2. Fann JI, Ingels NB, Craig Miller, D. 2008. *Pathophysiology of Mitral Valve Disease. Braunwald Cardiac Disease.* Chap. 41; 2008:974–1012.
3. Lillehei CW, Levy MJ, Bonnabeau RC. Mitral valve replacement with preservation of papillary muscles and chordae tendinae. *J Thorac Cardiovasc Surg.* 1964;47:532.
4. Ingels NB. Myocardial fiber architecture and left ventricular function. *Technol Health Care.* 1997;5:45-52.
5. Lower R. Tractatus de corde item De Motu and Colore Sanguinis et Chyli in cum Transitu. London, 1669;97-99.
6. Torrent-Guasp F. *Anatomia functional del Corazon.* Madrir: Paz Montalvo; 1957:628.
7. Buckberg G. Basic science review: the helix and the heart. *J Thorac Cardiovasc Surg.* 2002;124:863-883.

8. Anderson RH, Sanchez-Quitana D, Nierderer P, et al. Structural-functional correlation of the 3-dimensional arrangement of the myocytes making up the ventricular walls. *J Thorac Cardiovasc Surg.* 2008;136(1):10-18.
9. Pettigrew JB. On the arrangement of the muscular fibres in the ventricles of the vertebrate heart, with physiological remarks. *Philos Trans.* 1864;154:445-500.
10. Brachet JL. Sur le cause du movement de dilatation du Couer (dissertation). Paris: Imprimerie de Didot Jeune; 1813.
11. Hansen DE, Sarris GE, Niczyporuk MA, et al. Physiologic role of the mitral apparatus in left ventricular regional mechanics, contraction synergy and global left ventricular systolic function. *J Thorac Cardiovasc Surg.* 1989; 97:521.
12. Pitarys CJ, Forman MB, Panayiotou H, et al. Long-term effects of decision of the mitral apparatus on global and regional ventricular function in humans. *J Am Coll Cardiol.* 1990;89:132.
13. David TE, Burns RJ, Bacchus CM, et al. Mitral valve replacement for mitral regurgitation with and without preservation of chordae tendinae. *J Thorac Cardiovasc Surg.* 1984;88:718.
14. Horskotte D, Schulte HD, Bircks W, et al. The effect of chordal preservation on late outcome after mitral valve replacement: a randomised study. *J Heart Valve Dis.* 1993;2:150.
15. Rao C, Hart J, Chow A, et al. Does preservation of the sub-valvar apparatus during mitral valve replacement affect long-term survival and quality of life? A microsimulation study. *J Cardiotorac Surg.* 2008;3:17.
16. Lee EM, Shapiro LM, Wells FC. Importance of subvalvular preservation and early operation in Mitral valve surgery. *Circulation.* 1996;94(9):2117-2123.
17. Barlow CW, Imber CJ, Sharples LD, et al. Cost implications of mitral replacement versus repair in mitral regurgitation. *Circulation Supp II.* 1997;96(9):II90-II95.
18. Hansen De, Cahill PD, Derby GC, et al. Relative contributions of the anterior and posterior mitral chordae tendinae to canine global left ventricular systolic function. *J Thorac Cardiovasc Surg.* 1987;93:45.
19. Deniz H, Sokullu O, Sanioglu S, et al. Risk factors for posterior ventricular rupture after mitral valve replacement: results of 2560 patients. *Eur J Cardiothorac Surg.* 2008;34: 780-784.
20. Zegdi R, Carpentier A, Doguet F, et al. Systolic anterior motion after mitral valve repair: an exceptional cause of late failure. *J Thorac Cardiovasc Surg.* 2005;130(5): 1453-1454.
21. Barlow JB, Borman CK. Aneurysmal protrusion of the posterior leaflet of the mitral valve. An auscultatory-electrocardiographic syndrome. *Am Heart J.* 1966;71(2):166-178.
22. Feindel C, Tufail Z, David T, et al. Mitral valve surgery in patients with extensive calcification of the mitral annulus. *J Thorac Cardiovasc Surg.* 2003;126(3):777-781.
23. El-Amin WO, Thomson DS. *Heart Lung Circ.* 2006;15(21): 146-147.

When asked to write about *Barlow mitral valve*, some degree of unease and discomfort may rapidly rise. During the preparation phase when one thinks about the content and tries to organize it logically, one may be hit by a simple and iconoclastic question. What is a "Barlow mitral valve"? What does it mean? What is the most precise definition of the word?

Definition

The term "Barlow" is extensively used in the surgical literature, and some authors, reporting on some aspect of this specific etiology of mitral valve regurgitation, even use the word in the title of the article.[1-4] Unfortunately, in none of these references, there is a clear and undisputable definition or description of this very commonly used term.

The field of degenerative mitral valve regurgitation is difficult to define accurately because of the scarcity of basic work. If one concentrates on one pathological aspect recognizable during surgery namely the excess of tissue, clinical observation teaches us that this varies a lot from one patient to the other, in its location, its extent, and its severity and that there is a mosaic between rare patients with no visible excess of tissue and rare patients with generalized excess of tissue. To try to partially clarify the haze surrounding the term "Barlow," as it is used in the surgical community, let us list facts from the least disputable to the most adventurous use of this term.

John Barlow is a Cardiologist, born in 1924, who spent most of his professional life at the Cardiology Department of the University of Witwatersrand in South Africa. In 1963,[5] Barlow et al. published their landmark paper on the late systolic murmurs and clicks and related them to the mitral valve. Barlow et al. demonstrated mitral regurgitation on left ventricular cineangiocardiography in four patients who had murmurs confined to late systole.[6] Criley subsequently termed this condition mitral valve prolapse.[7] Based on surgical examination and pathological findings, Read[8] and Bittar[9] made the relation between late systolic clicks and murmurs, mitral insufficiency, and myxoïd degeneration. The first echocardiographic study of this valve anomaly was published by Shah[10] and the following "information explosion" relating to mitral valve prolapse has spread confusion in the terminology of degenerative mitral valve disease, each author using a new term: "myxomatous degeneration," "floppy leaflet," "mitral valve prolapse," "billowing leaflets," "Barlow disease," and so on.

John Barlow has always referred to this syndrome as the "Billowing mitral leaflet syndrome," avoiding the term prolapse. Similar to surgeons like Carpentier, Duran, or Yacoub, he restricted the use of this term to situations with a dysfunction of the mitral valve secondary to a failure of leaflet coaptation resulting in the displacement of an involved leaflet's edge.[11] Importantly, according to John Barlow, the "billowing mitral valve may be focal, involving only a portion of one scallop, usually the middle scallop of the posterior leaflet or it may be more advanced and diffuse.[11]"

Carpentier introduced the "Barlow's disease" when he made a clear distinction between the billowing mitral leaflet syndrome, now called Barlow's disease, and fibroelastic deficiency on the basis of

P. Perier
Department of Cardiovascular Surgery, Herz und Gefäss Klinik, Bad Neustadt/Saale, Germany
e-mail: pperier@club-internet.fr

R.S. Bonser et al. (eds.), *Mitral Valve Surgery*,
DOI: 10.1007/978-1-84996-426-5_7, © Springer-Verlag London Limited 2011

clinical patterns, echocardiographic findings, and gross features,[12] whereas only small differences were evident on qualitative histology.[13]

Authors reporting on surgical techniques or surgical results of "Barlow mitral valve" have difficulties to precisely define what the spectrum of their work is.[1-4] There are common characteristic features on which everyone would agree: marked billowing and excess of tissue can make the appearance of the mitral valve complex and worrisome making surgeons uneasy about the feasibility of valve repair. Degenerative mitral valve disease is a spectrum and the billowing and excess of tissue, as stated by Barlow himself, may be focal or extensive. Does a mitral valve with prolapse of two segments of the anterior leaflet and two segments of the posterior leaflet with billowing and excess of tissue of two third of the posterior leaflet and one third of the anterior leaflet belong to the so-called Barlow mitral valve? A mitral valve with a prolapse of the whole posterior leaflet showing severe excess of tissue and billowing and mucoid degeneration should probably not be classified as a "Barlow mitral valve," but may present a technical challenge equal to the one of a typical "Barlow mitral valve."

Instead of using ill-defined terms, which do not fit the everyday life and may obstruct our understanding, it would be more accurate and less speculative to use the same segmental classification to describe the mitral valve lesions as the one we use to describe dysfunctions. A valve could be described for example as a type II P2-P3/A2-A3 prolapse with P2-P3/A2-A3 billowing and excess tissue. Whatever the dysfunction, the etiology, and the lesions, a mitral valve becomes difficult to repair when more than three segments are prolapsed and show billowing and excess tissue, and this is what practically matters for the surgeon.

The difficulty of the operation comes from the extent of the prolapsed area, the amount of excess tissue, which poses a specific technical problem because it predisposes to the development of left ventricular outflow tract (LVOT) secondary to systolic anterior motion (SAM), and the thickness and irregularity of the leaflet tissue, which is due to the mucoid degeneration. Good understanding of the mitral valve and its interaction with the left ventricle is mandatory.

The operation will be described with four phases: valve assessment, choice of strategy, implementation of surgical techniques, and control of the result.

Valve Assessment

Valve analysis should be thorough and systematic using always the same algorithm. The valve analysis should be done using echocardiographic and surgical approaches.

Echocardiographic Analysis

The echocardiographic analysis should be meticulous. Lesions and dysfunctions are extensive so that one should take specific care to scanning and systematically analyze all the different segments of the valve, taking also the commissures into consideration. The echocardiographic analysis, however, may have some pitfalls. For example, in case of extensive prolapse of the posterior leaflet, there is no buttress for the anterior leaflet and the free edges of this leaflet may rise at an abnormal level close to or slightly above the annulus level (Fig. 7.1). In this situation, the question of whether the anterior leaflet is prolapsing may be raised.

Surgical Valve Analysis

Surgical analysis of the entire valvular and subvalvular apparatus should be performed systematically. The following parameters should be assessed: mobility of the free edge of the leaflets – excess of tissue – mucoid degeneration responsible for a decreased pliability and irregularities of the surface of the leaflet.

Free Edge Mobility

With the use of nerve hooks, the level of the free edge is compared to that of a "reference point" usually P1. Valve analysis should be careful, systematic, and performed in an organized way. Result of the surgical analysis should be compared to the echocardiographic analysis. In case of extensive prolapse of the posterior leaflet, echocardiography may detect a mild prolapse of the anterior leaflet because of its inability to coapt due to the lack of support from the severely prolapsing posterior leaflet as explained earlier. An accurate surgical analysis will show no difference between the

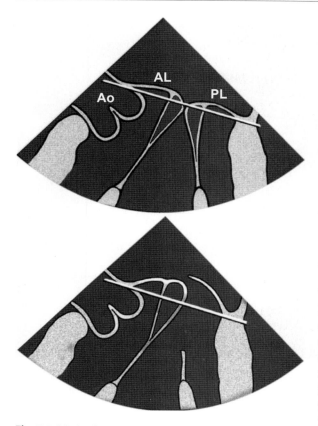

Fig. 7.1 Mechanism of bileaflet prolapse in patients with severe posterior leaflet prolapse and no anterior chordal rupture. (*top*) Normal anatomy, with leaflet coaptation occurring at the annular level, denoted by the solid line. (*bottom*) There is posterior leaflet flail due to chordal rupture. Anterior leaflet prolapse is caused by loss of posterior leaflet support at the zone of coaptation (From Gillinov et al.[14] Copyright Elsevier 1999)

during mitral valve repair because it predisposes, especially when affecting the posterior leaflet to the development of systolic anterior motion of the mitral valve.[15] When analyzing the posterior leaflet, one should evaluate not only the height of the posterior leaflet but also, more importantly, its width; the process of excess of tissue may transform for instance the normally quadrangular P into a trapezoidal element. At this point, it is critical to analyze the incisurae between the different scallops of the posterior leaflet. In these patients, they usually are very variable in their number and anatomy, being rarely almost nonexistent, most of the time deep and complex reaching the mitral annulus.

Mucoid Degeneration

The quality of the leaflet tissue should be examined. Excessive and exuberant myxomatous degeneration can render the leaflet irregular with bulging deformations, which may impair the quality of the surface of coaptation. Accumulation of myxomatous material at the base of the posterior leaflet may impair the mobility of the posterior leaflet at its hinge, and making it impossible to transform the posterior leaflet into a vertical buttress (Fig. 7.2).

The valve assessment may be time-consuming, but it is the most important step of the operation. A mistake, due to lack of good exposure, or a superficial analysis, will most likely lead to a poor repair. At the end of the valve analysis, the surgical strategy can be planned.

level of the reference point and the free edge of the anterior leaflet. As pointed out by Gillinov,[14] in this setting correction of posterior leaflet alone should result in restoration of normal valve function.

The lack of reliable reference point is a rare and complex situation. In such patients, the posterior leaflet should be treated first, and then a syringe bulb test should be performed to assess the result. Of course, if the test shows definite anterior leaflet prolapse, this should be corrected accordingly.

Excess of Tissue

Excess of tissue is one of the hallmarks of degenerative mitral valve disease and poses a specific challenge

Surgical Strategy

The goal of any valve repair is to restore the coaptation surface as conceptualized by Carpentier,[16] and to maintain it in the inflow region of the left ventricle, away from the outflow. A mitral valve repair may be difficult and demanding; nevertheless, it consists only of two steps: correct any abnormal leaflet motion and reshape and stabilize the annulus with ring implantation.

The issue of excess of tissue is a cornerstone of the operation because it has been recognized, especially when affecting the posterior leaflet, as a major risk factor for postoperative SAM,[15] which leads to a dynamic

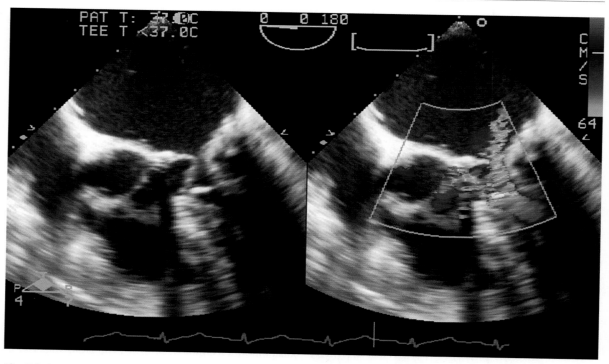

Fig. 7.2 Accumulation of myxomatous material at the hinge of the posterior leaflet prevents it from hanging vertically from the annulus. Consequently, the surface of coaptation is anteriorly displaced in the left ventricular outflow tract resulting in an SAM

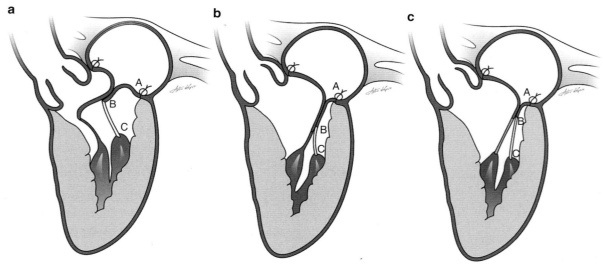

Fig. 7.3 (**a**) Dynamic left ventricular obstruction. (**b**) Situation avoided by maintaining the coaptation surface into the left ventricular inflow region using appropriately short chordae. (**c**) Same situation avoided by reducing the height of the posterior leaflet by a sliding plasty (AB = height of the posterior leaflet; B = free edge of the posterior leaflet; BC = length of the chordae) (From Perier et al.[29] Copyright Elsevier 2008)

left ventricular obstruction[17] (Fig. 7.3a). Subsequently, the first step and the most important will be the management of the posterior leaflet.

Because of the great variability of the dysfunctions and lesions, and of the quality of the leaflet tissue, it is impossible to recommend standardized techniques for the repair of this type of mitral valves. Nevertheless, it is necessary to follow a standardized strategy, a "road map" that will guide the choice of the techniques. This strategy will be driven by the goal that the reestablishment and the reconstruction of a large and posterior coaptation surface against which the anterior leaflet will come in apposition.

Repair of the Posterior Leaflet

Leaflet Mobility

Since leaflet tissue is the primary component of the coaptation surface, it is logical to preserve as much of it as possible. Leaflet resection followed by either plication annulus[18] or sliding leaflet plasty[19] has been associated with excellent long-term results.[20,21] However, a surgeon may face a myriad of questions during an operation such as "How large the resection should be?", "What if the prolapse is very extensive and involves more than one third of the posterior leaflet?", "Should an annulus plication with its subsequent deformation of the subannular area and the risk of kinking of the circumflex artery be performed to close the gap after resection?", or "Should a sliding plasty be performed to have a more regular distribution of stresses and minimize the risks of SAM because of the excess of tissue?" Moreover, posterior leaflet is typically composed of three different scallops of different heights.[22] The highest portion (P2 scallop) sustains the greatest stress during systole.[23] Instead of resecting leaflet tissue, our approach, "the respect rather than resect" (RRR) strategy, targets correction of leaflet prolapse, while preserving leaflet tissue to ensure a larger coaptation surface and a decrease in the stress.

Typically, echocardiographic results after mitral valve repair show a posterior leaflet with little or no mobility hanging vertically from the annulus and forming as shown experimentally[24,25] and clinically[26] a buttress against which the anterior leaflet comes into apposition. The goal of the operation is to intentionally achieve this specific aspect, to reconstruct a large, smooth, regular, and vertical surface of coaptation, and to avoid SAM.

In case of excess of tissue, SAM is due to an anterior displacement of the coaptation surface in the left ventricular outflow tract, as shown in Fig. 7.3a. In such a situation, the combined height of the posterior leaflet (AB) is too long, allowing the edge of the posterior leaflet (B) to enter the ventricular outflow tract. To avoid SAM, it is necessary either to reduce the height of the posterior leaflet (AB), that is to say to perform a sliding plasty whose goal is to precisely decrease the height of the posterior leaflet (Fig. 7.3c), or to decrease the length of the chordae (BC) (Fig. 7.3b). This can be achieved with the use of artificial chordae by adjusting their length so that the posterior leaflet will remain vertical, posterior, and parallel to the posterior wall of the left ventricle in the inflow region. The more excess of tissue there is, the shorter the chordae should be. This forms the basis of the principle of "respect rather than resect" (RRR) as it has been previously described.[27] The goal of RRR approach is to correct prolapse of the posterior leaflet without leaflet resection and typically uses CV-4 expanded polytetrafluoroethylene (Gore-Tex, W. L. Gore & Associates, Flagstaff, AZ) suture neochordae to resuspend the free edge of the posterior leaflet. To correct a P2 prolapse, two pairs of artificial chordae are implanted in the fibrous portion of each papillary muscle with a figure of eight suture and then brought through the free edge of the prolapsing posterior leaflet. The number and placement of the artificial chordae may vary according to the extent and the location of the prolapsed area; however, the basic architecture of the subvalvular apparatus must be respected.

The goal is to correct the prolapse and to transform the posterior leaflet into a smooth, regular, and vertical buttress parallel to the posterior wall of the left ventricle against which the anterior leaflet will come in apposition. Length of the artificial chordae is critical and determined to compensate for any excess tissue of the posterior leaflet so that its free edge cannot move anteriorly toward the left ventricular outflow tract, but remains in the left ventricular inflow. Schematically, if there is no excess tissue, the length of the artificial chordae is selected so that the free edge of the prolapsed area reaches the same level as the nonprolapsed reference point, usually P1. If there is excess tissue, the length of the artificial chordae is selected to bring the free edge of the prolapsed area to a lower level, typically 5–8 mm beneath the plane of the annulus, depending on the height of the posterior leaflet (Fig. 7.3b).

The Goal of a Smooth and Vertical Surface of Coaptation

A typical RRR approach without any leaflet resection may be preferred when quality and quantity of posterior leaflet tissue is adequate to achieve a smooth and regular coaptation surface. However, localized and limited leaflet resection may be required to reconstruct the posterior leaflet and transform it into a smooth and vertical element. The extent, location, and shape of the resection (triangular, quadrangular, or atypical) should be guided by anatomical considerations:

- Excessive and exuberant myxomatous degeneration can render the posterior leaflet irregular with bulging deformations that need to be resected to obtain a smooth and regular surface of coaptation.
- Excess tissue, affecting not only the height of the posterior leaflet, but more importantly its width, transforms the normally rectangular scallop (usually P2) into a trapezoidal element. The placement of the annuloplasty ring may result in folds of the posterior leaflet altering the coaptation surface smoothness. Again, a localized leaflet resection to reshape the posterior leaflet may be necessary in this scenario.
- Accumulation of myxomatous material at the base of the posterior leaflet should be removed, as it is likely to change shape and prevents the leaflet from hanging vertically, causing it to protrude anteriorly, thus increasing the risk of SAM.
- Calcifications of the annulus should be removed as proposed by Carpentier.[28]

To ensure a proper continuous and regular posterior buffer, care must be taken to look for and suture incisurae of the posterior leaflet, especially if they are deep.

It is to note that this step of treatment of the posterior leaflet is typically the strategy known as the "respect rather than resect," which has been published some years ago.[27] It may be applied of course, in case of isolated prolapse of the posterior leaflet, which represents the majority of patients presenting with degenerative mitral valve disease. Midterm results have been published with satisfactory durability.[29]

Intermediary Surgical Test

When the posterior leaflet has been treated and transformed into a smooth and vertical buttress, the mitral valve can be tested, even though an annuloplasty ring has not yet been performed. Usually, there is enough leaflet tissue to ensure a good closure of the valve. Saline is injected into the left ventricle, the competency and the line of closure of the mitral valve is analyzed to finalize the decision of the strategy for the anterior leaflet.

A lack of regurgitation, associated with a symmetrical line of closure, posterior, close to the hinge of the posterior leaflet reflects a good result of the repair. In this case, it is possible to proceed to the last step of the operation: sizing and implantation of a ring annuloplasty device.

A persistent regurgitation or an asymmetrical line of closure means that very likely there is prolapse of the anterior leaflet, which needs to be corrected prior to sizing of the annuloplasty ring.

Repair of the Anterior Leaflet

A prolapse of the anterior leaflet is repaired with the use of artificial chordae. Typically, CV-4 expanded polytetrafluoroethylene (Gore-Tex, W. L. Gore & Associates, Flagstaff, AZ) sutures are anchored in the fibrous portion of the papillary muscles with a figure of eight suture. The number of artificial chordae needed to be implanted depends on the extent of the prolapsed area. Approximately, three pairs of artificial chordae arising from one papillary muscle are necessary to resuspend half of the anterior leaflet. Artificial chordae are then passed through the free edge of the anterior leaflet to be resuspended. Optimal chordae height is achieved by intermittent testing valve competency with ventricular saline injections after the ring annuloplasty has been placed, the goal being a symmetrical line of closure of the mitral valve. It is extremely rare that the billowing of the anterior leaflet is so marked that a localized resection of the anterior leaflet is necessary.

Ring Annuloplasty

Ring annuloplasty is mandatory after repair of a degenerative mitral valve, because of the dilatation and deformation of the mitral annulus. The sizing of the ring is critical. The anterior leaflet should be unfurled with a right-angle clam, and a sizer should be placed on the anterior leaflet, so that its surface matches the surface area of the anterior leaflet. There is sometimes some discrepancy between the width of the sizer and the one of the anterior leaflet. The most important parameter is the height of the anterior leaflet. This means that the annuloplasty ring is true-sized to the anterior leaflet. Most valves with excess tissue are large and so if rings are true-sizes, one expects to implant larger rings (size 36 mm and above) for these patients.

Control of the Result

Surgical Control

The result of the repair is assessed intra-operatively by injecting saline into the left ventricular cavity with a syringe bulb. Criteria for a good repair are the following: no regurgitation, symmetrical line of closure, which runs parallel to the ring, and posterior line of closure very close to the ring, giving an idea that the surface of coaptation is posterior away from the left ventricular outflow tract. However, even a perfect surgical result as assessed intraoperatively with the arrested heart does not preclude an unsatisfactory result at echocardiographic control with unacceptable mitral regurgitation, usually secondary to SAM.

There are cases when injection of saline in the left ventricle is unable to properly fill the cavity, and develop intraventricular pressure, so that the mitral valve cannot close, presenting an aspect of residual prolapse of the anterior leaflet. Before starting to implement techniques to correct this "prolapse," a careful assessment of the situation is necessary. In case of doubt, it is reasonable to ignore this test and to proceed to the echocardiographic control.

Echocardiographic Control

Intra-operative echocardiography is the tool for quality control and when showing satisfactory repair, it allows the patients to be safely transferred to the intensive care with the confidence of having achieved good repair.

It has been shown that the use of intraoperative echocardiography is associated with a decreased risk of reoperation.[30] Four critical parameters have to be analyzed in a systematic way.

Ideally, the repaired mitral valve should be totally competent. The valve should be scanned from one commissure to the other, at 0°, 60°, and 120°. The height of the surface of coaptation should be measured (it should be at least 8 mm). In case of residual regurgitation, a careful analysis of the regurgitation should be performed; i.e. severity and location. In this latter matter, 3D color examination is an optimal tool. Schematically, a minimal regurgitation located between both leaflets, despite a satisfactory height of the surface of coaptation, counts for irregularities in the leaflet tissue, and could be accepted. Any other cause of mitral regurgitation should lead to surgical revision, i.e., slight persistent prolapse, leakage outside the surface of coaptation, etc.. Schematically, only minimal regurgitation (<grade 1) should be tolerated.

The dynamics of the mitral valve should be monitored and the outflow tract examined. The presence of an obstruction of the outflow tract due to systolic anterior motion of the mitral valve should lead to finding out its causes, i.e., excessive anterior mobility of the free edge of the posterior leaflet, or septal hypertrophy. Inotropic support should be avoided before performing intraoperative echo, and it should be stopped in case of SAP.

The function of the left ventricle should be analyzed globally and segmentally. An impairment of the contractility of the lateral or inferior wall should raise the possibility of an injury of the circumflex artery.

The aortic valve should be controlled to ensure that no aortic regurgitation has been created at the time of surgery.

Generally speaking, intraoperative echocardiographic control should not be considered by the surgeon as a judging foe; on the contrary, it represents a tool for quality control facilitating the admission of the patient to the ICU with a satisfactory result, a prerequisite to have a smooth and uneventful postoperative course, and improving the chances of having a long-lasting repair.

In cases operated minimally invasively, echo will guide the weaning off bypass by assessing the filling of the left ventricle.

Degenerative mitral valve regurgitation may be associated with technical difficulties due to the extent of the dysfunction and the excess of tissue, a risk factor for obstruction of the outflow tract of the left ventricle. Valve repair has been shown to be possible in almost 100% of the patients. This goal can be obtained with a strict strategy based on a thorough valve analysis and the implementation of efficient surgical techniques.

References

1. Fasol R, Mahdjoobian K. *Repair of mitral valve billowing and prolapse (Barlow): the surgical technique.* 2002:602-605.
2. Flameng W, Meuris B, Herijgers P, et al. Durability of mitral valve repair in Barlow disease versus fibroelastic deficiency. *J Thorac Cardiovasc Surg.* 2008;135(2):274-282.
3. Lapenna E, Torracca L, De Bonis M, et al. Minimally Invasive mitral valve repair in the context of Barlow's disease. *Ann Thorac Surg.* 2005;79(5):1496-1499.
4. Oc M, Doukas G, Alexiou C, et al. Edge-to-edge repair with mitral annuloplasty for Barlow's disease. *Ann Thorac Surg.* 2005;80(4):1315-1318.
5. Barlow JB, Pocock WA, Marchand P, et al. The significance of late systolic murmurs. *Am Heart J.* 1963;66(4):443.
6. Barlow JB, Bosman CK. Aneurysmal protrusion of the posterior leaflet of the mitral valve. An auscultatory-electrocardiographic syndrome. *Am Heart J.* 1966;71(2):166-178.
7. Criley JM, Lewis KB, Humphries JO, et al. Prolapse of the mitral valve: clinical and cine-angiocardiographic findings. *Br Heart J.* 1966;28(4):488-496.
8. Read RC, Thal AP, Wendt VE. Symptomatic valvular myxomatous transformation (the floppy valve syndrome): a possible forme fruste of the Marfan syndrome. *Circulation.* 1965;32(6):897-910.
9. Bittar N, Sosa JA. The billowing mitral valve leaflet: report on fourteen patients. *Circulation.* 1968;38(4):763-770.
10. Shah P, Bramiak R. Echocardiographic recognition of mitral valve prolapse (abstract). *Circulation.* 1970;42(Supp 3):111-145.
11. Barlow JB. Idiopathic (degenerative) and rheumatic mitral valve prolapse: historical aspects and an overview. *J Heart Valve Dis.* 1992;1(2):163-174.
12. Carpentier A, Chauvaud S, Fabiani JM, et al. Reconstructive surgery of mitral valve incompetence: ten-year appraisal. *J Thorac Cardiovasc Surg.* 1980;79(3):338-348.
13. Fornes P, Heudes D, Fuzellier JF, et al. Correlation between clinical and histologic patterns of degenerative mitral valve insufficiency: a histomorphometric study of 130 excised segments. *Cardiovasc Pathol.* 1999;8(2):81-92.
14. Gillinov AM, Cosgrove III DM, Wahi S, et al. Is anterior leaflet repair always necessary in repair of bileaflet mitral valve prolapse? *Ann Thorac Surg.* 1999;68(3):820-824.
15. Mihaileanu S, Marino JP, Chauvaud S, et al. Left ventricular outflow obstruction after mitral valve repair (Carpentier's technique). Proposed mechanisms of disease. *Circulation.* 1988;78(3 Pt 2):I78-I84.
16. Carpentier A. Cardiac valve surgery – the "French correction". *J Thorac Cardiovasc Surg.* 1983;86(3):323-337.
17. Maslow AD, Regan MM, Haering JM, et al. Echocardiographic predictors of left ventricular outflow tract obstruction and systolic anterior motion of the mitral valve after mitral valve reconstruction for myxomatous valve disease. *J Am Coll Cardiol.* 1999;34(7):2096-2104.
18. Carpentier A, Relland J, Deloche A, et al. Conservative management of the prolapsed mitral valve. *Ann Thorac Surg.* 1978;26(4):294-302.
19. Carpentier A. The sliding leaflet technique. *Le Club Mitrale Newsletter.* 1988;1:5.
20. Perier P, Stumpf J, Götz C, et al. Valve repair for mitral regurgitation caused by isolated prolapse of the posterior leaflet. *Ann Thorac Surg.* 1997;64(2):445-450.
21. Mohty D, Orszulak TA, Schaff HV, et al. Very long-term survival and durability of mitral valve repair for mitral valve prolapse. *Circulation.* 2001;104(12 Suppl 1):I1-I7.
22. Ranganathan N, Lam JHC, Wigle ED, et al. Morphology of the human mitral valve. II. The valve leaflets. *Circulation.* 1970;41(3):459-467.
23. Kunzelman K et al. Replacement of mitral valve posterior chordae tendineae with expanded polytetrafluoroethylene suture: a finite element study. *J Card Surg.* 1996;11(2):136-145. discussion 146.
24. van Rijk-Zwikker GL, Mast F, Schipperheyn JJ, et al. Comparison of rigid and flexible rings for annuloplasty of the porcine mitral valve. *Circulation.* 1990;82(5 Suppl):IV58-IV64.
25. Green GR, Dagum P, Glasson JR, et al. Restricted posterior leaflet motion after mitral ring annuloplasty. *Ann Thorac Surg.* 1999;68(6):2100-2106.
26. Cohn LH, Couper GS, Aranki SF, et al. Long-term results of mitral valve reconstruction for regurgitation of the myxomatous mitral valve. *J Thorac Cardiovasc Surg.* 1994;107(1):143-150. discussion 150–151.
27. Perier P. A new paradigm for the repair of posterior leaflet prolapse: respect rather than resect. *Oper Tech Thorac Cardiovasc Surg.* 2005;10(3):180-193.
28. Carpentier AF, Pellerin M, Fuzellier JF, et al. Extensive calcification of the mitral valve anulus: pathology and surgical management. *J Thorac Cardiovasc Surg.* 1996;111(4):718-729. discussion 729–730.
29. Perier P, Hohenberger W, Lakew F, et al. Toward a new paradigm for the reconstruction of posterior leaflet prolapse: midterm results of the "respect rather than resect" approach. *Ann Thorac Surg.* 2008;86(3):718-725.
30. Gillinov AM, Cosgrove DM, Blackstone EH, et al. Durability of mitral valve repair for degenerative disease. *J Thorac Cardiovasc Surg.* 1998;116(5):734.

How I Assess and Repair the Barlow Mitral Valve: The *Edge-to-Edge* Technique

Michele De Bonis and Ottavio R. Alfieri

Introduction

The main cause of mitral regurgitation (MR) in the western world is degenerative mitral valve disease, which usually leads to prolapse or flail of the posterior, anterior, or both leaflets. Mitral valve repair has become the treatment of choice of degenerative MR providing predictable and durable results in most patients.[1,2] The most favorable outcomes have always been reported with isolated prolapse of the posterior leaflet treated by a simple procedure like quadrangular resection and annuloplasty. On the other hand, less gratifying results and more demanding surgical techniques have been associated with correction of mitral regurgitation due to anterior leaflet or bileaflet prolapse.[3–6] To increase the feasibility of repair in those more difficult settings, a new surgical technique, named edge-to-edge, was introduced by our group more than 15 years ago. The basic principle of the edge-to-edge is that the competence of a regurgitant mitral valve can be restored with a functional rather than an anatomical repair. This can be obtained by suturing the free edge of the diseased leaflet to the corresponding edge of the opposing leaflet, exactly at the site where regurgitation occurs. When the regurgitant jet is located in the central part of the mitral valve, the application of the edge-to-edge technique produces a mitral valve with a double orifice configuration. In this case, the operation is conventionally defined as double orifice repair, and the two orifices can have similar or significantly different sizes depending on the extension and location of the suture performed.

On the other hand, when the regurgitant jet is located in the commissural area, the application of the edge-to-edge technique at this level creates a single orifice mitral valve with a relatively smaller area. This second instance is usually called paracommissural edge-to-edge. There are situations in which the regurgitant jet of the mitral valve is not a single one. Particularly, in the setting of Barlow's disease with severe bileaflet prolapse, for example, multiple regurgitant jets are usually found along the entire line of coaptation of the anterior and posterior leaflet. In this case, the edge-to-edge approximation of the middle scallop of the anterior and posterior leaflet (A2 and P2) allows the elimination of most of the mitral insufficiency while the residual smaller regurgitant jets are effectively corrected by the association of a ring annuloplasty.

The first edge-to-edge repair case was performed in 1991 and more than 1,500 published cases have been accumulated worldwide so far with the longest follow-up now being longer than 15 years. The technique is attractive because of its simplicity, reproducibility, and effectiveness in different settings. Indeed, due to its versatility, the edge-to-edge technique has been used for correction of mitral regurgitation due to different etiologies and mechanisms including bileaflet prolapse (Barlow's disease), anterior leaflet prolapse, and commissural prolapse. Functional mitral regurgitation (secondary to ischemic or idiopathic dilated cardiomyopathy) has also been treated in our institution by this approach although this will not be discussed in this chapter.

The Edge-to-Edge Technique for Bileaflet Prolapse in Barlow's Disease

In Barlow's disease, a myxomatous degeneration process involves all the components of the mitral valve

M. De Bonis (✉)
Department of Cardiac Surgery, San Raffaele University
Hospital, Milano, Italy
e-mail: michele.debonis@hsr.it

apparatus leading to generalized bileaflet prolapse, severe annular dilatation, and severe mitral insufficiency. The free edges of these myxomatous valves are often irregular, with an increased number of clefts (Fig. 8.1) and multiple regurgitant jets at Doppler echocardiography. To perform an anatomical reconstruction of a mitral valve affected by such a generalized disease, all the lesions identified at annular, valvular, and subvalvular level need to be addressed during a rather complex operation requiring long aortic cross-clamp times. This type of correction can certainly be performed successfully, but it does require a high level of expertise, is technically demanding, and is not easily reproducible. Alternatively, the edge-to-edge technique can be adopted. The advantage of this approach is that it is simple and easily reproducible allowing the effective treatment of multiple and generalized anatomical mitral defects with a single and well-standardized surgical act. In the presence of severe mitral regurgitation due to Barlow's disease and bileaflet prolapse, the edge-to-edge technique restores valve competence just by suturing the middle scallop of the anterior and posterior leaflet (A2–P2) followed by ring annuloplasty.

The purposes of the edge-to-edge technique in Barlow's disease are multiple and can be summarized as follows:

- Correcting leaflets' redundancy, which is usually predominant in the middle of portions of the valve, corresponding to the scallops A2 and P2.

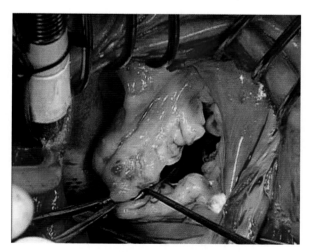

Fig. 8.1 Intraoperative view of a mitral valve affected by Barlow's disease with important redundancy of all the valve tissues, multiple scallops, chordal elongation, and severe bileaflet prolapse

- Forcing leaflets' coaptation by suturing together a segment of both leaflets and reducing the delay between the beginning of the ventricular contraction and valve closure in the regions of the mitral valve where the leaflets have not been stitched together.
- Eliminating leaflets' prolapse.
- Preventing postoperative systolic anterior motion (SAM), which is one of the common complications following the repair of the mitral valves affected by severe myxomatous degeneration of the leaflets.

Surgical Technique and Results

The edge-to-edge repair of the mitral valve is carried out through a conventional median sternotomy, although a minimally invasive small right thoracotomy can be used in selected cases. After conventional aortic and bicaval cannulation, total normothermic cardiopulmonary by-pass is established. Following aortic cross-clamping, cardioplegic arrest is obtained by delivering intermittent cold-blood cardioplegia into the ascending aorta whereas retrograde cardioplegia through the coronary sinus is associated only in the presence of aortic regurgitation. The interatrial groove is dissected and the mitral valve is approached through the left atrium. A careful inspection of the valve apparatus including annulus, leaflets, chordae tendineae, and papillary muscles represent the first and most important phase of any mitral repair procedure. In Barlow's disease, the mitral annulus is usually severely dilated, the leaflets are severely redundant due to the myxomatous degeneration process affecting their tissue, and multiple scallops are easily found. The entire valve is prolapsing, although the middle scallops of the anterior and posterior leaflets (A2 and P2) are usually the segments showing the most severe pathologic involvement. The chordae tendineae are significantly elongated and single or multiple chordal rupture can also be found causing one or more flailing lesions.

Once the presence of bileaflet prolapse has been established, a nerve hook is used to inspect the subvalvular apparatus and clearly identify the anatomical middle of the valve, which can be defined as the point of the anterior and posterior leaflets where the subvalvular structures converge. This region, corresponding approximately to the central part of the anterior and posterior leaflets, divides the mitral valve in two halves, each one connected by the underlying chordae tendineae to one papillary muscle. The chordae arising from the posteromedial papillary muscle and reaching the anterior leaflet are identified first (Fig. 8.2). Then, those arising from the anterior papillary muscle and reaching the anterior leaflet are recognized. The point of convergence of the groups of chordae on the anterior leaflet identifies the anatomical middle of the anterior leaflet (Fig. 8.3). The middle point of the posterior leaflet is then found in a similar

fashion. The first stitch of the edge-to-edge suture has to be positioned exactly in correspondence to this anatomical middle of the two leaflets (Fig. 8.4). This step is very important to avoid valve distortion and residual valve regurgitation. The symmetry of the two orifices created is immediately checked (Fig. 8.5). Two rows of suture are then passed along the whole length of the middle scallop of the anterior and posterior leaflets (A2 and P2) in correspondence to the rough zone: the first is a continuous mattress and the second is an over-and-over 4–0 polypropylene continuous suture (Fig. 8.6). The bites have to be rather deep, usually around 1 cm, to reduce the

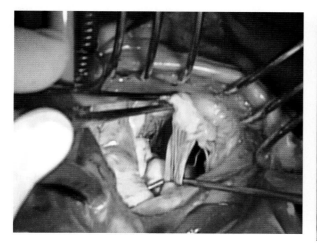

Fig. 8.2 The chordae connected to the anterolateral and posteromedial papillary muscles are recognized to identify the central portion of both leaflets

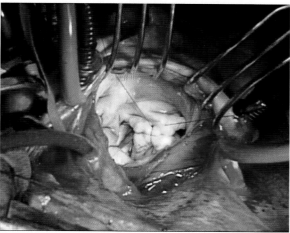

Fig. 8.4 A stay stitch is passed through the central part of A2 and P2 in correspondence to the rough zone and the symmetry of the two orifices created is checked

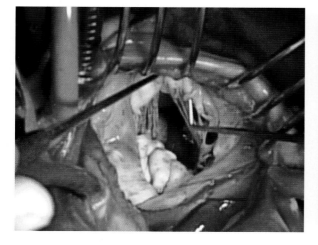

Fig. 8.3 The anatomical middle of the anterior leaflet is identified as the convergence point of the two groups of chordae

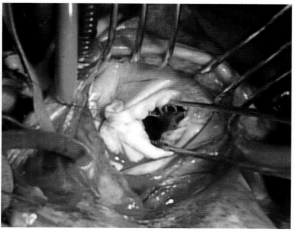

Fig. 8.5 View of the exact positioning of the first edge-to-edge stitch

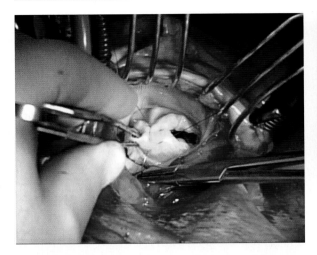

Fig. 8.6 The edge-to-edge suture is completed taking deep bites along the whole length of A2 and P2. A mattress followed by an over and over suture is performed through the rough zone of the leaflets

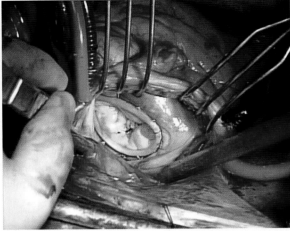

Fig. 8.7 After implantation of mitral annuloplasty semirigid ring, water testing shows optimal competence of the valve

height of the redundant leaflets and enhance the strength of the repair as much as possible. As a general rule, the more the redundancy present, the deeper the stitch should be. As far as the width of the suture is concerned, this should be minimized to reduce the risk of valvular stenosis. However, if valve prolapse and leaflet redundancy is severe, a wide suture, connecting the whole P2 free edge to the opposing A2, is usually necessary. In the presence of a flail segment, this has to be included in the edge-to-edge suture and the position of the stitch, in this circumstance, may be somewhat asymmetric, corresponding to the center of the flail portion of the leaflet. In this case, the size of the two orifices will be different, one being larger than the other one. Such an event should not raise any concern as far as both of them are competent and the sum of their areas is above 2.5 cm^2 for a normal size patient. A flexible or semirigid ring annuloplasty is always added to complete and stabilize the repair by remodeling the annulus and reducing its dimensions. The size of the ring is selected by measuring the inter-trigonal distance as well as the surface of the anterior leaflet. Once ring implantation has been completed, the final competence of the two mitral orifices is evaluated by forceful saline filling of the left ventricle (Fig. 8.7). If a residual leak is demonstrated, careful inspection of the repaired valve should be performed looking for possible clefts, which could be responsible for the persistence of regurgitation and which should be closed promptly.

The residual mitral area is assessed by direct inspection and, in case of doubts, Hegar valve dilators can be introduced into the orifices to be sure that a global valve area of at least 2.5 cm^2 in normal size patients has been left. Transesophageal echo-Doppler reassessment of the valve is routinely performed after weaning from cardiopulmonary by-pass. Typically, no residual mitral regurgitation is present and two diastolic flows can be visualized through the double orifice mitral valve. The valve area is commonly assessed by a planimetric method using the transgastric, short-axis view. Doppler methods can be used as well. Intraoperative pressure measurements of the transvalvular gradients may also be obtained to exclude mitral stenosis, although they are usually not necessary. Indeed, the potential risk of mitral stenosis is usually not an issue in Barlow's disease since, in most of these cases, preoperative valve area is excessively wide. The simplicity of the edge-to-edge technique makes it possible to repair complex Barlow's disease mitral valve with very short cross-clamp times. In our experience, mean cardiopulmonary by-pass and aortic cross-clamp times were 54 ± 13.8 min and 39 ± 6.7 min, respectively. Excluding patients undergoing associated cardiac procedures, mean cardiopulmonary by-pass and ischemic times were 47 ± 9.1 min and 33 ± 3.9 min.

Our experience with the edge-to-edge technique for the surgical treatment of bileaflet prolapse in the context of Barlow's disease includes 618 consecutive patients submitted to mitral valve repair from 1991 to

2007. Hospital mortality was 0.9%. Actuarial survival at 5 years was 93% ± 3.7% and freedom from reoperation 91% ± 3.2% with no patients requiring late reoperation for mitral valve stenosis. Echocardiographic follow-ups show good results of the repair, with stable competence and no progression of valve stenosis: the mean mitral valve area, assessed in a subgroup of 82 patients, was 10.2 ± 2.1 cm² preoperatively, decreased to 3.7 ± 0.8 cm² after repair, and did not significantly change at follow-up remaining 3.6 ± 0.97 cm².[7] Considering the unfavorable anatomical features and the complexity of the mitral valve lesions of patients affected by Barlow's disease, we consider these results very satisfactory.

In some patients with myxomatous degenerative disease of the mitral valve, the pathologic process involves mainly the anterior leaflet rather than the posterior one. In this case, an isolated anterior leaflet prolapse or flail may be found intraoperatively. Similarly, it is not unusual that one of the two commissural areas appear to be affected much more than the remaining portions of the valve, with the regurgitant jet localized in correspondence to the anterior or, more commonly, posterior commissure. In both situations, the edge-to-edge technique can still be conveniently used to effectively restore the competence of the valve, although with limitations, which will be detailed later. Indeed, our experience with the edge-to-edge technique in the presence of anterior leaflet or commissural lesions has been very satisfactory.

The Edge-to-Edge Technique for Anterior Leaflet Prolapse

We have analyzed and reported the late outcome of a series of 133 patients with segmental prolapse of the anterior leaflet submitted to isolated edge-to-edge repair and mitral annuloplasty over a period of 10 years.[8] No hospital deaths occurred and long-term (up to 13 years) clinical and echocardiographic follow-up was 100% complete. Overall, 10-year survival was 91% ± 4.06%, freedom from cardiac death 95.8% ± 2.83%, and freedom from reoperation 96% ± 2.3% with 93.2% of the patients being in NYHA functional class I or II at a mean follow-up of 4.5 ± 3.12 years (range 1 month to 13.2 years). The mean mitral valve

area after repair was 2.6 ± 0.6 cm² (range 2–4 cm²) and the mean mitral gradient 3.1 ± 1.5 mmHg (range 1.8–5.8 mmHg). Mitral stenosis was never detected immediately after surgery or later and, at the last follow-up, mitral regurgitation was absent or mild in 120 patients (90.1%), moderate in 10 patients (7.5%) and severe in 3 patients (2.2%). All these 3 patients were reoperated. These results were comparable to those obtained in our institution with patients submitted to standard quadrangular resection for prolapse of the posterior leaflet, which means that, in our experience, the edge-to-edge repair has been able to neutralize the prolapse of the anterior mitral leaflet as an incremental risk factor for suboptimal results in mitral valve repair. These results were obtained in patients with segmental prolapse of the anterior leaflet, involving only one scallop. On the other hand, in the presence of an extended anterior leaflet prolapse, involving more than one scallop, the edge-to-edge technique alone may not be sufficient to obtain a perfectly competent valve since a long suture would be required with higher risk of inducing mitral stenosis. Under the above circumstances, the implantation of artificial chordae may be required to eliminate incompetence without excessively reducing the mitral valve area.

The Edge-to-Edge Technique for Commissural Prolapse

Effective repair of prolapsing or flailing lesions of the commissural area of the mitral valve can be very challenging. The edge-to-edge technique associated to annuloplasty can enable a rapid and reliable mitral reconstruction and may be applied to correct either one or both leaflet prolapses/flails at the commissure. At the Cleveland Clinic, more than 100 patients with commissural prolapse/flail have been treated with suture closure of the commissure, with no instances of mitral stenosis, suture dehiscence, or recurrent prolapse in the follow-up.[9] Since 1998, our group has employed the edge-to-edge technique for approximation of the mitral valve leaflets at the commissural area in 115 patients for managing isolated commissural prolapse or flail with very satisfactory clinical and echocardiographic results.[10] The predictability and durability of repair have been demonstrated not only by the low incidence of reoperations (2 out of 114 hospital survivors, 1.7%) but also by the lack of recurrence of significant mitral regurgitation over time. In our series, an echocardiographic follow-up was performed in 108 patients at a mean postoperative time of 2.3 ± 1.9 years (median 2.0 years, range 1–8.3 years). Mitral regurgitation was absent in 60 patients (55.6%), mild in 43 (39.8%), moderate in 3 (2.8%), and severe in 2 (1.9%, both reoperated on). No instance of mitral stenosis was ever documented as indicated by the low transvalvular gradients recorded echocardiographically. The longest follow-up is now approaching 9 years and the satisfactory echocardiographic data obtained so far are certainly encouraging a strategy of early mitral repair also in the difficult setting of commissural mitral valve incompetence. In our opinion, commissural edge-to-edge repair associated to annuloplasty is probably the simplest and most reproducible method to repair commissural lesions. Because of its excellent clinical and echocardiographic result, it remains the method of choice to correct isolated commissural prolapse or flail at our Institution.

The Minimally Invasive Approach Option

In patients with severe mitral regurgitation due to Barlow's disease, an early surgery policy is nowadays recommended whenever a very high probability of repair can be ensured. Those patients are often asymptomatic and understandably reluctant to undergo a major operation through a median sternotomy. On the other hand, a minimally invasive approach through a small right thoracotomy is much more accepted and often specifically requested. The edge-to-edge technique, because of its technical simplicity and reproducibility, can be easily applied through a minimally invasive approach,[11] particularly in young patients, with good LV function and no significant comorbidities. Patients are intubated with a double-lumen endotracheal tube and a 14 F cannula is placed percutaneously through the right jugular vein into the superior vena cava. A 6- to 8-cm minithoracotomy is then performed through the fourth intercostal space and a soft tissue retractor is used for spreading the ribs. One port is created laterally to the incision to introduce both a 5-mm video scope and a CO_2 line to flush the operative field. Pericardial stay sutures are

passed through and fixed out of the chest. Following cannulation of the femoral vessels, cardiopulmonary bypass (CPB) is established between femoral artery and femoral and jugular veins, at 28°C–30°C. Aortic cross-clamp is performed by using the Chitwood transthoracic clamp inserted through the second or third intercostal space and intermittent antegrade cardioplegia is delivered through an aortic root catheter. The mitral valve is exposed in all cases through a left atriotomy using a transthoracic atrial retractor positioned in the fourth intercostal space. The valve is analyzed and repaired by direct vision through the minithoracotomy incision. Whenever the view is suboptimal, the inserted camera is used to improve valve assessment and reconstruction. Long-shafted Heartport instruments, passed through the minithoracotomy, allow suture placement, annuloplasty ring implantation, and knot tying. Complex prolapse in Barlow's disease can be effectively corrected through such a right minithoracotomy by using the edge-to-edge technique. Our clinical and echocardiographic data show a 100% freedom from reoperation and a stable competence of the mitral valve up to 4 years of follow-up. In our experience, the durability of the repair has never been compromised or jeopardized by the minithoracotomy access and the level of patient satisfaction in terms of cosmetic results, postoperative pain, and time to full recovery after the operation has always been very high. These results certainly justify the adoption of this strategy whenever considered feasible and, in particular, in a selected group of young and active people.

Edge-to-Edge Repair and Annuloplasty

At the beginning of our experience, the edge-to-edge technique has been adopted in some cases without an associated annuloplasty, particularly in old patients with severe mitral regurgitation and heavily calcified annulus. However, with increasing experience, it has been demonstrated that the lack of annuloplasty is one of the most important factors of edge-to-edge repair failure with a freedom from reoperation at 5 years, which decreases from 92% in patients with annuloplasty to 79% in those without.[12] One of the explanations of the necessity of concomitant ring annuloplasty in edge-to-edge repair has been reported by Timek and coworkers[13] who demonstrated that the tension on the edge-to-edge suture is dependent on the mitral annulus size. This means that if a further dilatation of the mitral annulus takes place after surgery, recurrent MR is likely to occur after edge-to-edge repair. Therefore, nowadays, we always recommend addition of an annuloplasty to the edge-to-edge repair, if technically feasible. The annuloplasty, besides increasing the coaptation surface of the leaflets and enhancing the competence of the valve, reduces the stress on the edge-to-edge suture and prevents the possibility of subsequent annular dilatation with positive effects on the long-term durability of the repair.

Double Orifice Edge-to-Edge Repair and Hemodynamics

When the edge-to-edge technique is adopted as a double orifice repair, the morphology of the mitral valve becomes that of a valve with two orifices. During the early phase of adoption of this technique, several concerns were formulated regarding the possible hemodynamic effects of such an unusual configuration on ventricular filling. A higher risk of thromboembolic complications was also postulated due to the increased turbulence of the diastolic flow through two mitral orifices rather than one. Clinical experience and computational model studies, however, have subsequently demonstrated that the hemodynamic performance of a double-orifice mitral valve is comparable to that of a single-orifice one of equivalent effective orifice area and the supposed increased risk of thromboembolic events has never been confirmed in clinical practice. The mitral hemodynamic depends exclusively on the total valve area and on the cardiac output[14] and not on the double-orifice shape. In double-orifice valve configuration, the velocity of the flow through each orifice is very similar to the one observed through a single-orifice valve of area equal to the sum of the areas of the two orifices. Moreover, the flow velocities through the two orifices are exactly the same, even when the orifice sizes are significantly different, which means that the Doppler sampling of any of the two orifices is sufficient to assess the hemodynamic of the mitral valve. Our clinical experience confirms these findings: in a series of 10 patients previously submitted to

double-orifice repair, the velocities recorded at each orifice by Doppler examination did not differ by more than 5% in sinus rhythm.

Edge-to-Edge Repair and the Risk of Functional Mitral Stenosis

Some concerns have been raised regarding the potential restrictive effect of the edge-to-edge technique during exercise.[15] In our experience, the gradients measured at rest across the mitral valve after edge-to-edge repair have always been very low, both immediately after surgery and at follow-up.[16] Moreover, to assess if the edge-to-edge mitral repair could be a limiting factor for exercise tolerance, we performed an exercise echocardiographic study in patients previously submitted to central double orifice mitral repair.[17] This study has clearly demonstrated that during physical exercise, the mean transmitral gradient after double-orifice mitral valve repair remains below 5 mmHg and the peak transmitral gradient does not exceed 10 mmHg. Moreover, the pulmonary pressure does not increase up to pathologic levels. Finally, the mean planimetric mitral valve area at peak of the stress is more than $4 \, cm^2$ coupled with hemodynamic physiologic response with a significant increase in stroke volume. According to those findings, it is possible to state that the artificially created double-orifice valves follow a physiologic behavior under stress conditions, with a good valvular reserve in response to the increased cardiac output. Functional mitral stenosis does not develop either at baseline or under exercise also with concomitant ring annuloplasty. Similar findings have been reported by other authors. Frapier and coworkers[18] have compared patients operated on either by Carpentier's techniques or by the edge-to-edge repair. Rest and exercise echocardiogram along with cardiorespiratory testing with maximal oxygen uptake were performed. At baseline, the mean mitral valve area was $2.5 \, cm^2$ after the edge-to-edge and $2.9 \, cm^2$ following classic mitral repair techniques ($p = 0.0018$). However, despite the higher mitral valve area reduction, the edge-to-edge technique did not induce more transvalvular gradients than classical Carpentier's repair. Indeed, mean mitral gradients at rest were not significantly different between the two groups, being 3.8 mmHg in the edge-to-edge and 3.3 mmHg in the classic techniques group, respectively. Moreover, at peak exercise, increase in the mitral gradient and maximum oxygen uptake (VO_2 max) was comparable between the two groups. This shows that the edge-to-edge repair is no more restrictive at peak exercise than classic repairs and provides the same efficiency on mitral regurgitation reduction and the same exercise tolerance as in Carpentier's techniques.

In conclusion, following the pioneering work of Carpentier,[19] the surgical armamentarium of mitral valve repair has been expanded over the years and predictable and durable results have been documented worldwide. The conservative treatment of mitral regurgitation due to Barlow's disease remains one of the most challenging situations for the cardiac surgeon. The introduction of the edge-to-edge technique has provided an additional contribution to the treatment of mitral regurgitation due to global myxomatous degeneration of the mitral valve. This simple technical solution has significantly increased the rate of mitral repair in patients with Barlow's disease in the surgical community. Over the years, the edge-to-edge technique has shown to be reproducible and durable in bileaflet prolapse (Barlow's disease), anterior leaflet prolapse, and mitral regurgitation due to commissural lesions. Simplicity, reliability, and effectiveness are the main advantages of the edge-to-edge technique and have led to its increasing widespread application in the surgical community.

References

1. Yun KL, Miller DC. Mitral valve repair versus replacement. *Cardiol Clin*. 1991;9:315-327.
2. Olson LJ, Subramanian R, Ackermann DM, et al. Surgical pathology of the mitral valve: a study of 712 cases spanning 21 years. *Mayo Clin Proc*. 1987;62:22-34.
3. Gillinov AM, Cosgrove DM, Blackstone EH, et al. Durability of mitral valve repair for degenerative disease. *J Thorac Cardiovasc Surg*. 1998;111:734-743.
4. Braunberger E, Deloche A, Berrebi A, et al. Very long-term results (more than 20 years) of valve repair with Carpentier's techniques in nonrheumatic mitral valve insufficiency. *Circulation*. 2001;104(12 Suppl 1):I8-I11.
5. Mohty D, Orszulak TA, Schaff HV, et al. Very long-term survival and durability of mitral valve repair for mitral valve prolapse. *Circulation*. 2001;104:I-1-I-7.
6. Flameng W, Herijjers P, Bogaerts K, et al. Recurrence of mitral valve regurgitation after mitral valve repair in degenerative valve disease. *Circulation*. 2003;107: 1609-1613.
7. Maisano F, Schreuder JJ, Oppizzi M, et al. The double-orifice technique as a standardized approach to treat mitral regurgitation due to severe myxomatous disease: surgical technique. *Eur J Cardiothorac Surg*. 2000;17:201-205.
8. De Bonis M, Lorusso R, Lapenna E, et al. Similar long-term results of mitral valve repair for anterior compared with posterior leaflet prolapse. *J Thorac Cardiovasc Surg*. 2006; 131(2):364-368.
9. Gillinov AM, Shortt KG, Cosgrove DM 3rd. Commissural closure for repair of mitral commissural prolapse. *Ann Thorac Surg*. 2005;80:1135-1136.
10. Lapenna E, De Bonis M, Sorrentino F, et al. Commissural closure for the treatment of commissural mitral valve prolapse or flail. *J Heart Valve Dis*. 2008;17:261-266.
11. Lapenna E, Torracca L, De Bonis M, et al. Minimally invasive mitral valve repair in the context of Barlow's disease. *Ann Thorac Surg*. 2005;79(5):1496-1499.
12. Alfieri O, Maisano F, De Bonis M, et al. The double-orifice technique in mitral valve repair: a simple solution for complex problems. *J Thorac Cardiovasc Surg*. 2001;122:674-681.
13. Timek TA, Nielsen SL, Lai DT, et al. Mitral annular size predicts Alfieri stitch tension in mitral edge-to-edge repair. *J Heart Valve Dis*. 2004;13:165-173.
14. Maisano F, Redaelli A, Pennati G, et al. The hemodynamic effects of double-orifice valve repair for mitral regurgitation: a 3D computational model. *Eur J Cardiothorac Surg*. 1999; 15:419-425.
15. Borghetti V, Campana M, Scotti C, et al. Preliminary observations on haemodynamics during physiological stress conditions following double orifice mitral valve repair. *Eur J Cardiothorac Surg*. 2001;20:262-269.
16. Maisano F, Torracca L, Oppizzi M, et al. The edge-to-edge technique: a simplified method to correct mitral insufficiency. *Eur J Cardiothorac Surg*. 1998;13(3):240-245.
17. Agricola E, Maisano F, Oppizzi M, et al. Mitral valve reserve in double-orifice technique: an exercise echocardiographic study. *J Heart Valve Dis*. 2002;11(5):637-643.
18. Frapier JM, Sportouch C, Rauzy V, et al. Mitral valve repair by Alfieri's technique does not limit exercise tolerance more than Carpentier's correction. *Eur J Cardiothorac Surg*. 2006;29:1020-1025.
19. Carpentier A. Cardiac valve surgery. The French correction. *J Thorac Cardiovasc Surg*. 1983;86:323-327.

How I Assess and Repair the Barlow Mitral Valve

Francis C. Wells

From a practical point of view, there are two groups of patients with degenerative mitral valve disease. The largest group presents with localized mural leaflet prolapse, usually as a result of a ruptured chord, localized to the postero-inferior portion of that leaflet (Fig. 9.1).

This is the group that Carpentier categorized as having a deficiency or lack of fibro-elastic tissue within the leaflets and chords.[1] Repair of these valves is relatively straightforward and there are a number of methods to accomplish this satisfactorily. Most of them can be adequately dealt with by a well-trained general cardiac surgeon. They are not for further discussion here.

The second group, those that are the subject for discussion here are referred to as being of the Barlow's[2] type and consist of patients with a much more complex lesion. The concept of aneurysmal protrusion of mitral leaflets was described by Barlow in 1966.[3] His paper was written at a time when cardiac ultrasound did not exist and all clinical observations relied on expert clinical examination and, in particular, clever interpretation of auscultation and the then-evolving electrocardiogram. The observations described therein reflected the wise use of considerable clinical expertise, something that is becoming scarce in the modern era of cardiology. Subsequent analysis revealed that this excessive leaflet tissue with multiple areas of prolapse could affect both the aortic and mural leaflets of the valve. This has been referred to as a billowing of the mitral valve leaflets. It is usually associated with a very large valve orifice and chronic worsening mitral valve regurgitation. We are fortunate that modern cardiac ultrasound examination clearly reveals the characteristics of

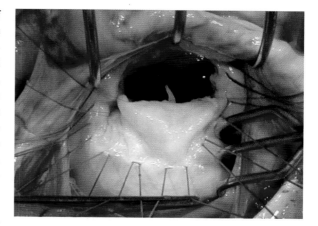

Fig. 9.1 Isolated prolapse of mural leaflet of the mitral valve with ruptured chord

these valves such that they can always be distinguished prior to surgery. This structural distinction allows the referral of the patient with this problem to an experienced cardiac surgeon well versed in the necessary techniques to successfully repair such valves. This is very important for the benefit of the patient as the repair rate for Barlow's valves is inferior to that for simple mural leaflet prolapse.[4] Of perhaps even greater concern however is the number of patients in whom repair has been attempted and in whom the result is unsatisfactory leaving the patient with significant residual regurgitation or systolic anterior motion of the aortic leaflet giving rise to left ventricular outflow obstruction.[4] These outcomes are likely to be worse than prosthetic valve insertion with subvalve preservation.

The orifice of Barlow valve is much larger than those with other forms of regurgitation. The circumference of Barlow's valve may be as much as 50–100% larger than a normal valve for someone with a similar body surface area. The anterior leaflet alone often has

F.C. Wells
Department of Cardiac Surgery, Papworth Hospital, Cambridge, Cambridgeshire, UK
e-mail: francis.wells@papworth.nhs.uk

R.S. Bonser et al. (eds.), *Mitral Valve Surgery*,
DOI: 10.1007/978-1-84996-426-5_9, © Springer-Verlag London Limited 2011

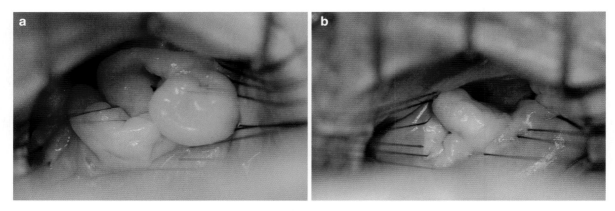

Fig. 9.2 (**a**) The excessive leaflet tissue with interchordal billowing. The thickening and yellowing of the tissue of the leaflets can be appreciated. (**b**) The excessively tall mural leaflet can be seen

a surface area that is greater than the whole of the valve with fibro-elastic deficiency. The condition is defined by the presence of multiple areas of leaflet prolapse affecting both aortic and mural leaflets. The prolapse is more as a result of massive excess of leaflet surface area between chordal attachments than chordal lengthening or rupture (although both exist in the Barlow's valve), giving an appearance that Carpentier referred to as "billowing" (Fig. 9.2).

Significant lengthening of multiple chords is seen. Strangely chordal rupture is less frequent (Fig. 9.3). Chords are often variably thickened and may fuse to the ventricular wall themselves and may calcify, a process that often extends into the atrio-ventricular junction and down into the basal ventricular muscle.

The excess leaflet tissue that is found between chordal attachments, which gives rise to the billowing segments, is thickened and on microscopic examination can be seen to have lost the normal architecture. Myxomatous material infiltrates the tissue causing it to become architecturally amorphous and structurally thickened (Fig. 9.4).

These pathological changes appear to weaken the leaflet structure allowing the interchordal leaflet to stretch and hence to billow[6]; an appearance that is abundantly clear on ultrasound visualization (Fig. 9.5).

The anatomical disposition of the papillary muscles within the ventricle often does not conform to the standard pattern. Frequently, the chords arise from multiple smaller papillary projections, and the papillary muscles may be partly or wholly fused to the ventricular wall. In some cases, the chords appear to arise directly from the ventricular wall. This arrangement is usually found at the postero-medial commissure with the

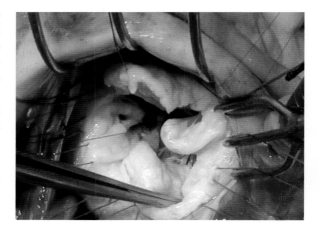

Fig. 9.3 This image reveals the multiple clefts that are to be found in a Barlow-type valve along with the chordal elongation and rupture of a chord to the aortic leaflet. The thickening and fusion of the chords to the mural leaflet can also be seen

antero-lateral papillary muscle conforming to the more usual pattern.

A feature that appears to be common to this type of valve, and whose consequence is infrequently commented upon, is the apparent atrialization of the origin of the mural leaflet, which is accompanied by an upward and outward motion of the base of the left ventricle in mid-late systole.[5] This appears to be as a result of the elongated chords and papillary muscles giving rise to a lack of coaptation of the leaflets. Thus, during late systolic contraction of the base of the ventricle and the papillary muscles, the absence of leaflet coaptation, through loss of the normally complete atrio-ventricular loop (see Chap. 6), causes the ventricular muscle in mid-cavity to move toward itself and that at

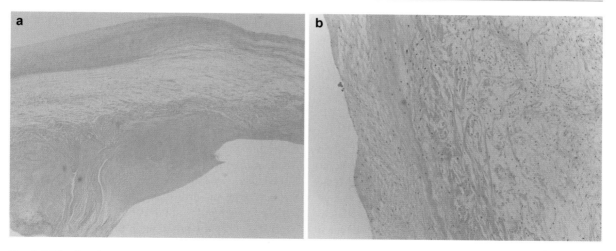

Fig. 9.4 Histology images showing the thickened and myxomatous leaflets found in a Barlow patient

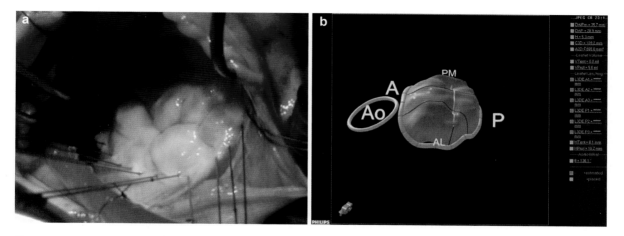

Fig. 9.5 These images reveal the billowing leaflets in reality and in three-dimensional echo format

the base to move outwards and upwards. This abnormal motion exaggerates valve orifice dilatation. This abnormal motion is completely corrected when the chordal attachments are corrected to a normal length and a good length of coaptation has been restored.

When the valve is inspected at the time of surgery, the leaflets often look as though their origin has rolled up onto the atrial wall. There is often a gutter found running along the annulus and the tissue is yellowed and thickened. Blood may have infiltrated these tissues, and it is the site for calcification, which may spread down into the ventricular muscle. It rarely if ever seems to spread into the atrial wall. Sometimes, a white material emanates from the subendocardium in this region when annular sutures are placed at this point. This is likely to be the early stage of calcification.

All these features make the task of reconstruction of the normal function of this type of valve challenging for the inexperienced surgeon. It can be argued that these valves should only be taken on by reference mitral valve surgeons to allow the highest rate of reconstruction.[6] Most reported series continue to report repair rates of less than 80% for this group of patients.[7] There is, however, an argument, which has not properly been tested in the context of a randomized prospective trial, that valve insertion with complete subvalve preservation in these patients is the equal of repair and may even be superior in some groups of patients and certainly in the hands of many surgeons can be made. The most important contribution in this area is a recently published propensity matched study of repair versus replacement from the

Cleveland Clinic in which patients receiving prosthetic valves fared just as well as those in the repair group.[8]

Valve Assessment

Although, as Barlow and others demonstrated,[9] there are distinct auscultatory features to be heard in patients with Barlow's valves, for all practical purposes today this is an echocardiographic diagnosis and assessment. All the features described above can be very well demonstrated by this means. Indeed, with the advent of near-real time 3-D echocardiography, it is possible to generate images that are almost as distinct as seeing the actual valve[10] (Fig. 9.6).

Moreover, if the valve is to be repaired, the complexities of this type of valve disorder are such that clear images of the moving, working valve are indispensible for complete planning of the procedures that will be necessary to restore them to satisfactory function.

The first thing to be said in the description of the assessment of Barlow's valve applies to all valves. That is that full assessment should be carried out with as near normal loading conditions for the valve as possible. The determination of the timing for surgical intervention relies on the quantification of regurgitation, atrial and ventricular size, and dynamic function. For a full picture, studies should be carried out following exercise as well as at rest to mimic the reality of the patient's life.

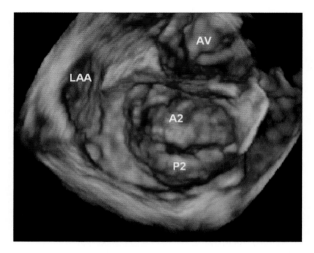

Fig. 9.6 A three-dimensional image of a Barlow valve shown from the surgeon's perspective

It is unwise to revise a planned surgical procedure at the time of surgery. Proper pre-operative work-up is superior in every way to an on-table assessment when the cardiac loading conditions are abnormal. The anesthetized patient will usually have been deprived of oral sustenance for at least 6 and often up to 12 h. Circulating volume will have been depleted and the anesthetic drugs reduce peripheral vascular resistance. Therefore, the true functional significance of the valve disorder cannot be safely determined. Even the use of intravenous volume loading and pressure loading through inotropic drugs cannot reproduce the natural state. In other words, on-table trans-esophageal assessment should not be relied upon to derive all information that is necessary to make the appropriate surgical decisions.

In my practice, patients are assessed using precordial ultrasound for initial assessment preferably with studies completed at rest and on exercise. These studies derive the necessary physiological information. Many so-called "asymptomatic" patients will complain of symptoms on a degree of exercise that is unusual for them or exhibit signs of physiological cardiovascular stress when exercised on a treadmill. Others will have experienced symptoms until commenced on medical therapy and when asked on treatment omits to confess to pretreatment symptoms.

Trans-esophageal ultrasound with 3-D assessment adds to the surgical anatomical knowledge of the valve. In some cases, cardiac magnetic resonance imaging (MRI) will be used to derive information about contractile reserve. Cardiac computed tomography (CT) is particularly useful in assessing annular calcification as well as coronary status.

I use the following parameters to decide on the timing of surgery. In the so-called asymptomatic patient, the presence of severe mitral regurgitation accompanied by any increased left ventricular diastolic volume, adjusted for body surface area that is above normal parameters, surgery is indicated in the hands of the experienced mitral valve surgeon. By the nature of Barlow's disease, by the time such patients are identified, many will also have an increase in left ventricular end systolic volume (LVESV). The encroachment of increased LVESV suggests the beginning of irreversible ventricular change. The presence of paroxysmal atrial fibrillation is another such indicator. It is my opinion, supported by evidence, that to delay surgery in this setting simply increases the likelihood of persistent postoperative ventricular dysfunction.[11,12]

Symptomatic patients with severe mitral regurgitation should be offered surgery directly. Well-timed intervention will minimize the risks of surgery while increasing the likelihood of repair and a satisfactory long-term result.

On the other hand, ultra-early intervention by inexperienced surgeons resulting in an unnecessary valve replacement should be avoided. Thus, the timing of surgery has to be integrated with access to an appropriately skilled surgeon. Both these factors are written in the American guidelines for the timing of surgery in patients with mitral regurgitation.[13,14] These guidelines gave a class 1 recommendation to mitral valve surgery for chronic severe mitral regurgitation (MR) in the presence of symptoms, a left ventricular ejection fraction of less than 60% (difficult to assess in the presence of severe MR with varying loading conditions!), and end-systolic dimension of more than 40 mm. Mitral valve repair was recommended over replacement for most patients (class 1 recommendation). The guidelines advise that such persons be referred to surgical centers at which surgeons are experienced in mitral valve repair. The European guidelines are very similar but differ over the recommendation for surgery in asymptomatic patients where it remains level 1 in the European guidelines but is level 2A in the American guidelines.[15]

The details of the morbid anatomy of the valve can be further examined and defined on the operating table with trans-esophageal ultrasound. As mentioned above, the advent of "near"-real-time 3-D images has significantly enhanced the ability to reveal the detail of the lesions that are to be found.

For the purpose of repair, the most important information is the following:

- The site and direction of the regurgitant jet. Obviously, these areas will be the initial target for repair. There may be more than one point of regurgitation or there may be a broad front suggesting a degree of annular dilatation in addition to the localized anatomical distortion. Often, there will be an area of significant leak but with multiple other areas of varying coaptation height and leaflet billowing. The direction of the jet will reveal which leaflet is overriding the other. If the jet is directed toward the mural leaflet and the posterior wall of the left atrium, then the aortic leaflet is overriding the mural one. If the jet is in the opposite direction, then the reverse is true. A central jet indicates bileaflet prolapse as well as annular dilatation.

- The depth of coaptation of the leaflets and the areas of distinct prolapse.

- The chordal arrangement and, if the ultrasound equipment is sophisticated enough, the papillary muscle array and their relationship within the ventricular cavity.

- The presence of displacement of the mural leaflet toward the left atrium and the motion of the mural annulus. If the leaflet is very tall and there is significant backward rotation of the leaflet associated with the appearance that the leaflet origin is more from the atrial wall, this may be an indication for leaflet detachment and reattachment to the true atrioventricular junction. This may involve the resection of a sliver of mural leaflet at its tallest part to reduce its height.

- The presence, circumferential extent, and depth of any annular calcification. This ought to have been recognized before surgery and a Cardiac CT scan would have delineated the extent of the problem quite accurately (Fig. 9.7). If it is very extensive, it may call into question the operability of the lesion. The decision to decalcify the annulus will usually have been made in advance of the operation.

- Several measurements of the mitral orifice and leaflet height are useful. The septo-lateral, inter-commissural diameters, and the circumference of the mitral orifice are important when deciding on the

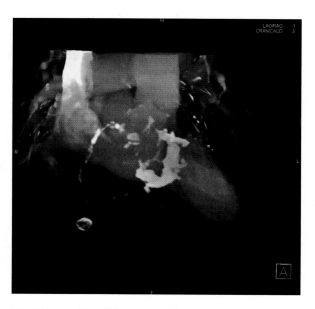

Fig. 9.7 A cardiac CT image revealing extensive calcification in the atrio-ventricular junction and extending into the ventricular myocardium

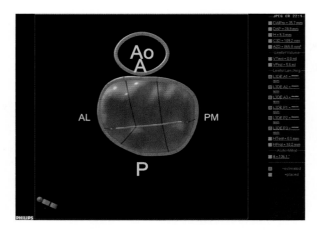

Fig. 9.8 A left atrial three-dimensional image of the mitral valve using software that allows quite accurate measurement of the annular circumference and septomural and intercommissural distances

choice of the size of any annuloplasty ring selection (Fig. 9.8).

- The lengths of the mural and aortic leaflets and the ratio of their heights are important measurements in minimizing the risk of producing abnormal systolic anterior leaflet motion (SAM) and thereby left ventricular outflow tract obstruction. How these measurements are utilized will depend on the degree of annular dilatation that may be present. This can be determined in turn by looking at the residual coaptation height and the breadth of the regurgitant jet. Overreduction of the mitral orifice will increase the risk of producing SAM, especially if the mural leaflet is greater than 40% of the height of the aortic leaflet.

From the information listed above, it is possible to build a good mental picture of the valve prior to opening the heart.

Surgical Exposure

In all forms of surgery, good exposure of the part to be operated upon is essential for a successful outcome and in the pursuance of perfection. This is particularly true in the reconstruction of this complex form of mitral pathology. There are many small steps that can be taken which add up to optimal exposure. My personal approach is as follows:

The patient is positioned supine on the operating table with a support placed longitudinally between the shoulder blades under the upper part of the back. This projects the thorax forwards and the arms fall back somewhat from the sides of the chest. The patient is centered on the table so that there will be adequate room at the upper end for the surgeon to work freely. The correct positioning of the operating theater light is also important. These maneuvers are the surgeon's responsibility and should not be left to others. I use a median sternotomy and will not discuss the role of minimal access surgery here.

Once the sternum has been opened, I suspend both sides of the incised pericardium beneath the edges of the sternal retractor to elevate the whole heart as far as possible. Cannulation for cardio-pulmonary bypass involves two uncrossed transatrial cannulae, one into each vena cava. If the intercaval distance is short, then a metal-tipped right-angled cannula placed directly into the superior vena cava and another at the cavo-atrial junction will release more space for surgical access. Once on cardio-pulmonary bypass, I use a left ventricular vent, both for optimal drainage of the left ventricle and the evacuation of air from the ventricle at the end of the procedure. The heart is arrested using blood cardioplegia delivered in ante-grade fashion. Myocardial protection is further augmented with a pericardial circulation of saline at 4°C, and intermittent cardioplegia administration every 20-30 min throughout the time of aortic cross-clamping.

With the heart arrested, both venae cavae are snared with nylon tape and the snares elevated as far as possible to draw the interatrial groove as high as possible.

The interatrial groove is then developed by separating the atria as far as possible. The left atrium is then incised. The inferior wall is sutured to the parietal pericardium along with a further suction catheter placed between the pulmonary veins. This allows a very dry operative field and excellent vision throughout the procedure. The left atrial retractor is then introduced. I favor a self-retaining retraction system. This gives the best stability to the exposure and allows the assistant (trainee) to focus on the operative procedure. It is important to note that after a few minutes, the heart muscle will relax more than in the first instance and the retraction can be increased by careful further traction on the retractor blades. The surgeon should not hesitate to re-arrange the retractor blades at any time in the operation to give the maximum exposure. With this

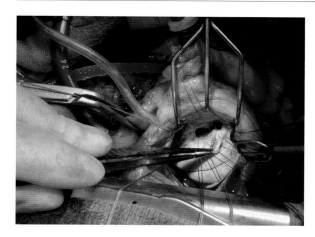

Fig. 9.9 An intra-operative photograph showing the surgical setup and exposure for the mitral valve

approach, it is rare indeed that a good view of the mitral valve cannot be obtained (Fig. 9.9).

Even at this stage, however, further improvement in exposure can be gained. The mitral valve lies in a plane that is oblique to the surgeon when seen from the usual point of view through the left atrium. The antero-lateral commissure falls away posteriorly and, often, is difficult to visualize without help. Fortunately, patients with this condition usually have significant atrial enlargement, which improves the available exposure. In addition, the leaflets usually crowd together and their proper relationship cannot be seen on first inspection. For this reason, my next step is to place the annuloplasty sutures around the annulus from trigone to trigone omitting the intertrigonal septal portion. This allows the whole valve to be brought into the same plane and gives excellent exposure.

The final assessment of the valve can then be carried out. By this time, the surgeon will have a multidimensional image of the valve in mind. It is now time to test this knowledge on the actual valve structures. Injection of cold saline under pressure across the valve until the root of the aorta can be seen to be pressurized will allow the overall structure of the valve to be inspected. This maneuver will usually reveal the prolapsing segments of the valve. The placement of the annuloplasty sutures will already have produced some reduction in the annular orifice and that is often enough to reduce the amount of regurgitation such that the line of coaptation can be painted with a sterile marker pen. The highest points of prolapse can also be marked with the pen. When the ventricular cavity is then emptied,

the coaptation line can be seen on each leaflet margin. This will also reveal the degree of prolapse from one segment to another. More detailed analysis can then be performed using a pair of nerve hooks and comparing the height of the aortic and mural leaflets with one another and with itself at each point along the valve.

Next, the arrangement of the papillary muscles is carefully inspected. The length and character of the chords is assessed, particularly those associated with the areas of prolapse. The presence of chordal fusion to themselves or to the ventricular wall is noted as is the presence of any calcification. It should now be clear what will be required to restore competence.

As described earlier, Barlow's valve by definition has multiple areas of prolapse along with areas of leaflet billowing, which may not be associated with lack of coaptation. Although chordal rupture is less common than in fibro-elastic deficiency if present, it is noted and factored into the repair. The presence of ruptured chords can deflect the inexperienced surgeon from other areas of less obvious but equally important defects. Commissural prolapse involving aortic and mural leaflets is common and often involves both commissures.

It cannot be stressed enough that this time spent in analysis is the most important time in the procedure. From these observations, the optimal strategy for repair can be devised.

Strategies for Surgical Repair

There are two diametrically opposed strategies that can be adopted. The first and perhaps still the most widely accepted involves the resection of the worst areas of leaflet prolapse coupled with annular reduction techniques. The second is an approach wherein the areas of prolapse are corrected by the construction of new chords using suture material, which most commonly is Gore-Tex. This preserves all the available surface area of leaflet tissue, which in turn reduces the stress within the leaflets. Although the resultant leaflet surface area is larger, some orifice reduction and stabilization is needed to address the orifice dilatation caused by ventricular dilatation. With this philosophy, the size of annuloplasty ring that is needed is inevitably larger than in cases where leaflet surface area has been reduced by resection and should be based on the whole orifice area of the valve. With resectional techniques, the selection of annuloplasty ring size tends to be based on the surface area of the aortic leaflet and the intertrigonal distance.

My personal experience has been that although the resectional approach gives a satisfactory result for many Barlow's valves, it cannot always allow a satisfactory result, especially when there are multiple lesions that must be corrected. Once the resections have been carried out, it is impossible to restore the status quo, and if the valve's function is unsatisfactory, valve replacement is the only recourse. Whereas, when neo-chords are used, if the initial result is not acceptable, then they may be removed and an alternative approach can be used. As a result of this experience, I set out to restore competence by retaining all valve tissue and reconstructing the natural state with new chords.

The first stage then is to establish how many points of leaflet prolapse there are and whether one leaflet is responsible or are both prolapsing beyond the plane of the annulus. I then mark each point of prolapse at its apex with a fine polypropylene stitch. I then reduce the segments of mural leaflet prolapse first. The appropriate papillary muscle head is identified and the suture with small Teflon pledgets is placed through the junction of the fibrous tip with the muscular bulk. Three throws are placed on the stitch, which is then held on a rubber shod clip. This is repeated with as many sutures as are needed (Fig. 9.10).

Each of the sutures is then placed through the apogee of each of the prolapsed segments of the leaflet.

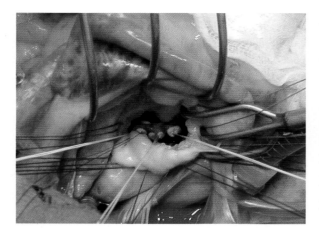

Fig. 9.10 Teflon pledgeted 4'0' Gor-Tex sutures placed through the papillary muscle heads ready for placement in the mural leaflet edge

The stitch is passed twice through the leaflet from the ventricular side. The leaflet edge is then pulled down to the appropriate height to give correct apposition. The chordal length that has been measured prior to opening the heart may be of some use and some operators prepare the neo-chordal length in loops prior to the operation.[16] With experience, however, it is possible to judge the correct height with relative ease. Once all the sutures are in place and at the correct length, they are tied to secure the length. This can be achieved by passing each end of the suture around the pair of sutures from each direction. With this technique, once the knot has been tied, it will be drawn beneath the coaptation line of the leaflet. Other techniques have been described such as the formation of a simple suture loop at the point of fixation on the leaflet and then to pass the suture through this loop and tie it at the papillary muscle end.[17]

For aortic leaflet repair, further chords are attached to the papillary muscles at the appropriate points, but this time using the anterior end of the papillary muscle crescent. If the prolapse is central, then I place chords from each of the papillary muscle heads to give extra strength and to balance the support. Once again, the leaflet is drawn down to the appropriate coaptation point. To achieve this, I imagine the plane of the working valve and draw the edge up to 1 cm below this point, as this will give the appropriate degree of leaflet coaptation. Mural leaflet coaptation is then achieved by the appropriate reduction in annular orifice size with the choice of annuloplasty ring. Once again, in this setting the ring is sized on the surface area of the whole orifice and not just the aortic leaflet surface area. If only the aortic leaflet is used to size the orifice, then this is more likely to lead to the deflection of the aortic leaflet into the outflow tract by the mural leaflet producing SAM, as in this disease the mural leaflet is often disproportionately tall (Fig. 9.11).

Even when the primary approach is to create new chords, there will be circumstances where resection and reconstruction may improve the result. If the surgeon chooses to adopt resectional techniques, then the preliminary assessment remains the same. Excessive areas of billowing between the chords to either the aortic or mural leaflet may be dealt with by small triangular resections (Fig. 9.12).

If the surface area of the valve is to be kept in proportion to the natural orifice, then the depth of resection in the aortic leaflet should not extend too far into the body of the leaflet, as that will reduce its overall surface area leading to coaptation problems with the mural leaflet at either end of the commissural line and will introduce abnormal stress patterns within the leaflet.

If quadrangular or triangular resection is to be used to resolve all of the mural leaflet problems, then they need to be multiple. As the mural leaflet is often excessively long, for a satisfactory result with resection and to prevent SAM, it is necessary to reduce the height of the leaflet. When using leaflet resection, the orifice of the valve will need to be reduced significantly to allow proper coaptation. This can be accomplished in the process of mural leaflet reduction by sliding annuloplasty. On completion of the repair, the mural leaflet ought to be no more than one third of the height of the aortic leaflet.

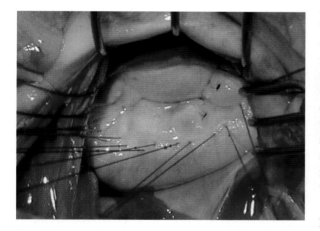

Fig. 9.11 The valve shown in Figs. 9.2a and 9.5a following repair with neo-Gor-Tex chords

However, this process can place the aortic leaflet at risk of being compressed. This can give rise to insufficient central coaptation. Thus, an alternative approach is a more radical triangular excision of the aortic leaflet, which extends to the annulus. This must then be matched by a mural leaflet quadrangular resection based on imaginary radial lines dropped from the top dead center of the aortic annulus along with a sliding mural annuloplasty so that the resection margins can be rotated toward each other producing no tension on any point of the new lines of apposition.[18] I have not found it necessary to use such a radical resection and prefer to direct corrective surgery to the specific individual lesions.

No discussion of repair techniques for valves with severe bileaflet prolapse is complete without description of the creation of the double orifice valve as described by Alfieri.[19] The concept was first triggered by the finding of a naturally bileaflet valve in which the central portion of the aortic and mural leaflets was fused. The apposing edges of leaflets at the point of worst prolapse are sutured together in two layers first at the leading edge and then at the level of the secondary chords over a length of 1–2 cm. The need to support this type of repair with a circumferential annuloplasty ring is unclear in patients with Barlow's disease. If the surgeon chooses to implant an annuloplasty ring, then it must be sized on the whole circumference of the valve and will rarely be less than a size 35 ring.

Excessive atrialization (retroversion of the hinge point into the left atrium) of the mural leaflet with excessive leaflet height may be corrected by detachment of the leaflet from the atrio-ventricular junction

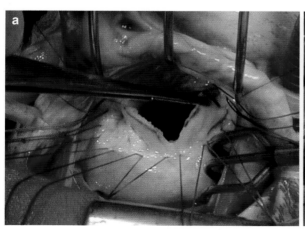
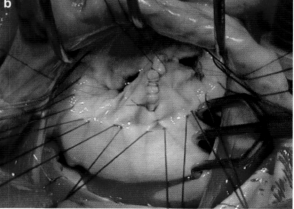

Fig. 9.12 These intra-operative photographs show a triangular resection of excess tissue in the mural leaflet of the mitral valve

with resection of some leaflet tissue from its base. The leaflet is then reattached further into the valve orifice with a continuous suture. However, my experience has shown that the same objective can be achieved with neo-chords. Simply by restoring a good coaptation and full valve competence, in the final stages of systolic contraction the papillary muscle shortening draws the leaflets down into the ventricle and the base of the heart moves inwards and downwards in the correct way. In this situation again, it is most important not to reduce the orifice of the valve greatly as SAM will result.

Occasionally, after all the major corrections have been accomplished, there may remain some commissural prolapse at the junctions of the aortic and mural leaflets. This is often correctable with lateral Alfieri-type stitches or a Carpentier "magic" stitch to imbricate these areas. Extreme commissural prolapse here may also be

corrected by lateral commissuroplasty. To achieve this, the excess leaflet is excised in quadrangular fashion and the lateral edge of the aortic leaflet undermined and detached from the annulus. Similarly, the mural leaflet is detached. Plication sutures can then be placed through the denuded annulus to eradicate the gap. The mural leaflet can then be slid inside the aortic leaflet and the two edges sewn back together and the reunited leaflet sewn to the annulus over the area of plication thus forming a new lateral commissure (Fig. 9.13).

Calcification, even if it is extensive, can be dealt with as previously described (in chapter on MV insertion with subvalve preservation by F Wells). The detached mural leaflet can then be reattached (Fig. 9.14).

Although there is little data on the long-term outcome of these techniques, specifically in the Barlow's valve sub-type of mitral valve leaflet prolapse, I have found

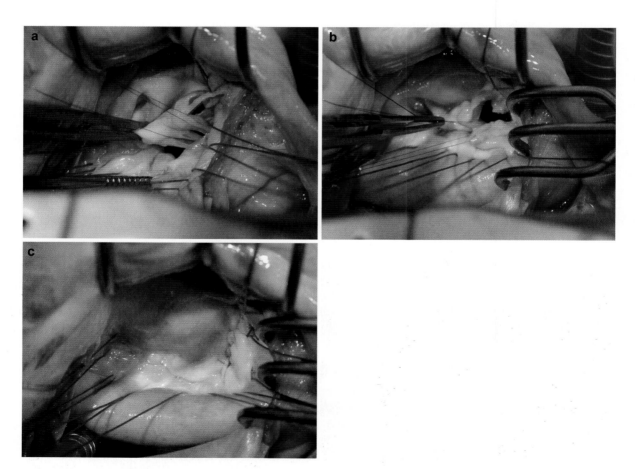

Fig. 9.13 These three photographs show a severe commissural prolapse (**a**), a quadrangular resection of the prolapsing segment of both aortic and mural leaflets (**b**), followed by the completed repair by sliding "plasty" (**c**)

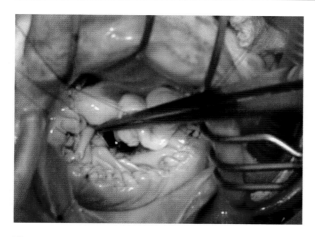

Fig. 9.14 The atrio-ventricular junction has been decalcified and reconstructed with a bovine pericardial patch. The detached mural leaflet is in the process of being reattached

that if the valve is completely competent at the end of the procedure with a good height of coaptation all along the commissures of the aortic and mural leaflets, then good long-term function can be anticipated. Any remaining unresolved valve regurgitation can be expected to result in further problems in the years to come.

References

1. Carpentier A. Cardiac valve surgery – The "French Correction. *J Thorac Cardiovasc Surg.* 1983;86(3):323-337.
2. Barlow JB, Pocock WA. Billowing, floppy, prolapsed or flail mitral valves? *Am J Cardiol.* 1985;55:501-502.
3. Barlow JB, Bosman CK. Aneurysmal protrusion of the posterior leaflet of the mitral valve. *Am Heart J.* 1966; 71(2):166-178.
4. Adams DH, Anyanwu AC. Seeking a higher standard for degenerative mitral valve repair: begin with etiology. *J Thorac Cardiovasc Surg.* 2008;136(3):551-556.
5. Adams D, Anayanwu A. Seeking a higher standard of repair for degenerative mitral valve repair: begin with aetiology. *J Thorac Cardiovasc Surg.* 2008;136(3):551-556.
6. Anyanwu AC, Adams DH. Etiologic classification of degenerative mitral valve disease: Barlow's disease and fibroelastic deficiency. *Semin Thorac Cardiovasc Surg.* 2007;19:90-96. Elsevier Inc.
7. Flameng W, Meuris B, Herijgers P, Herregods MC. Durability of Mitral valve repair in Barlow's disease versus fibroelastic deficiency. *J Thorac Cardiovasc Surg.* 2008; 135:274-282.
8. Gillinov AM, Blackstone EH, Nowicki ER, et al. Valve repair versus valve replacement for degenerative mitral valve disease. *JTCVS.* 2008;135(4):885-893.
9. Barlow JB, Pocock WA, Marchand P, et al. The significance of late systolic murmurs. *Am Heart J.* 1963;66:443-452.
10. Hoole SP, Liew TV, Boyd J, Wells FC, Rusk R. Transthoracic real-time three-dimensional echocardiography offers additional value in the assessment of mitral valve morphology and area following mitral valve repair. *Eur J Echocardiogr.* 2008;9:625-630.
11. Lee EM, Shapiro LM, Wells FC. Importance of subvalvar preservation and early operation in mitral valve surgery. *Circulation.* 1996;94(9):2117-2123.
12. Enriquez-Sarano M, Avierinos J-F, et al. Quantative determinants of the outcome of asymptomatic mitral regurgitation. *NEJM.* 2005;352(9):875-884.
13. American College of Cardiology, American Heart Association Task Force on Practice Guidelines. ACC/AHA 2006 guidelines for the management of patients with valvular heart disease: a report of the American associations; developed in association with the Society of Cardiovascular anaesthesiologists endorsed by the Socity of Thoracic surgeons. *J Am Coll Cardiol.* 2006; 48(3):e1-e148.
14. Bonow RO, Carabello BA, Chatterjee K, et al. Focused update incorporated into the ACC/AHA 2006 guidelines for the management of patients with valvular heart disease: a report of the American College of Cardiology/American Heart Association Task Force on Practice Guidelines (Writing Committee to revise the 1998 guidelines for the management of patients with valvular heart disease): endorsed by the Society of Cardiovascular Anaesthesiologists, Society for Cardiovascular Angiography and Interventions and Society of Thoracic Surgeons. *J Am Coll Cardiol.* 2008; 52(!£):e1–e142.
15. Vahanian A, Baumgartner H, Bax J, et al. Guidelines on the management of valvular heart disease: The task force on the Management of Valvular Heart Disease of the European Sociaty of Cardiology. *Eur Heart J.* 2007; 28:230-268.
16. Seebuger J, Borger MA, Falk V, Mohr FW. Gore-Tex© loop implantation for Mitral valve prolapse: The Leipzig loop technique. *Op Tech Thorac Cardiovasc Surg.* 2008; 13(2):83-90.
17. Dang N, Stewart AS, Kay J, et al. Simplified placement of multiple artificial mitral valve chords. *Heart Surg Forum.* 2005;8(3):E129-E131.
18. Fasol R, Mahdjoobian K. Repair of mitral valve billowing and prolapse (Barlow): the surgical technique. *Ann Thorac Surg.* 2002;74:602-605.
19. Maisano F, Schreuder FF, Oppizzi M, Fiorani B, Fino C, Alfieri O. The double orifice technique as a standard approach to treat mitral regurgitation due to severe myxomatous disease: Surgical technique. *Eur J Cardiothorac Surg.* 2000;17:201-205.

Ischemic Mitral Regurgitation

10

Robert J.M. Klautz and Robert A.E. Dion

Introduction

Definitions and Mechanisms

Ischemic mitral regurgitation (IMR) is a functional problem, which results from ischemia of the ventricle. Except in the case of ischemic papillary muscle rupture, the mitral apparatus is anatomically normal and the regurgitation is solely caused by abnormal systolic motion of the ventricle, interfering with the normal closure physiology of the valve. This is an important precision as organic mitral valve disease can simply be concomitant to coronary artery disease: in this situation, the prognosis is usually much better than in IMR. To make the situation even more complex, IMR can aggravate a pre-existent organic disease. Precise echocardiographic diagnosis is therefore needed to distinguish the different components and consequences of the underlying disease process.

Normal closing physiology of the mitral valve involves the synchronization of different parts of the heart: the mitral annulus, the mitral leaflets, the subvalvular apparatus, including chordae tendineae and papillary muscles, and finally the ventricle itself (Figs. 10.1a and b). In IMR, the ventricular dysfunction is the predominant problem: for the normal mitral valve to close, it is imperative that the apex moves toward the base of the heart, relieving the tension on the subvalvular apparatus and allowing the leaflets to close. More precisely, both papillary muscles are simultaneously moving inward and upward during systole. The abnormal motion of the ventricle in the case of IMR can be very subtle. It can be caused not only by ischemia-induced absence of contractility of parts of the ventricle (Fig. 10.1b) but also due to dyssynchronic contraction.[1,2] It can be related to an infarct scar or to a dysfunctional but viable myocardium. The severity of IMR is less related to the amount of dysfunctional myocardium than to its influence on the function of the subvalvular apparatus. The infero-posterior area of the left ventricle is particularly important in this respect and also small infarcts in this area can cause severe mitral regurgitation (MR). On the other hand, even large anterior myocardial infarcts can have little impact on the closing mechanism of the mitral valve. It is surprising that dysfunction of the papillary muscles alone, except ischemia-induced severe elongation, are not a cause of MR.[3-5]

Another important feature of IMR is its dynamic character. In situations of increased circulatory volume or during exercise, the MR can easily increase. Conversely, after diuretic treatment, after afterload reduction, and under resting conditions, MR can be markedly reduced. Under anesthetic conditions, the MR can even be completely absent, even though it was graded severe before operation. This dynamic nature can very well explain the dyspnea that some coronary patients experience instead or on top of their angina. Rather than considering this as a form of equivalent angina, one should echocardiographically evaluate these patients, preferably under exercise conditions.[6]

Consequences of Ischemic Mitral Regurgitation

The impact of IMR on the outcome is dramatic. Enriquez-Sarano showed that in the chronic phase

R.J.M. Klautz (✉)
Department of Cardiothoracic Surgery, Leiden University Medical Center, Leiden, The Netherlands
e-mail: r.j.m.klautz@lumc.nl

R.S. Bonser et al. (eds.), *Mitral Valve Surgery*,
DOI: 10.1007/978-1-84996-426-5_10, © Springer-Verlag London Limited 2011

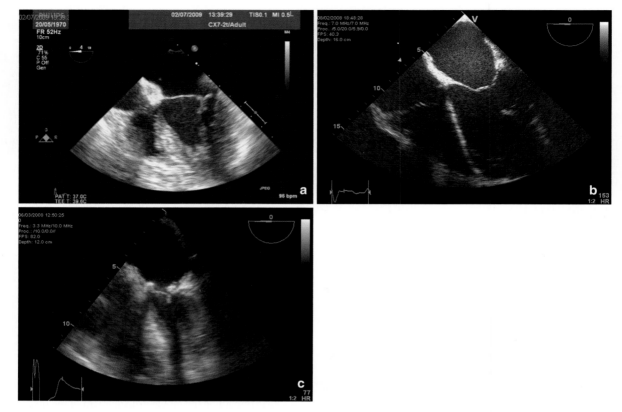

Fig. 10.1 (**a**) Echocardiographic view of normal mitral valve closure (end-systolic frame); (**b**) echocardiographic view of restrictive mitral valve closure (end-systolic frame) due to enlargement of the left ventricle. Note the tenting of the mitral valve and small length of coaptation; (**c**) echocardiographic view after restrictive mitral annuloplasty (end-systolic frame). Note the increased length of coaptation compared to Fig. 10.1b

after myocardial infarction, the presence of IMR is associated with excess mortality, independent of baseline characteristics and degree of ventricular dysfunction (Fig. 10.2).[7] The mortality risk was directly related to the degree of IMR as defined by effective regurgitant orifice (ERO) and regurgitant volume (RV).[8] Based on the impact on survival, IMR was already defined as severe if ERO > 20 mm² and RV > 30 mL, which are half of the values used to define severe degenerative MR. Even more, an exercise-induced increase in MR has also shown to be a predictor of mortality and hospital admission for heart failure.[9] It is not difficult to understand why MR in the setting of a reduced ventricular function has such an impact on outcome. The chronic volume load imposed on a ventricle that already has reduced reserve capacity leads to further remodeling. The above-mentioned dynamic nature makes it difficult to estimate the exact burden

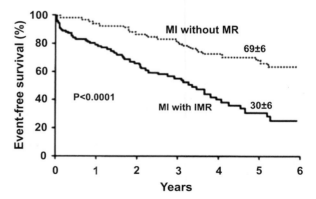

Fig. 10.2 Survival free of congestive heart failure or cardiac death (event-free survival) in asymptomatic patients after myocardial infarction (MI) according to the presence (*continuous line*) or absence (*dotted line*) of ischemic mitral regurgitation (IMR) at diagnosis. The event-free survival rates at 5 years are indicated ± the standard error. With permission from Grigioni et al.[7]

of a given degree of IMR as this may vary during the day. But let us take an example; suppose ejection fraction is 50% and the regurgitant volume is 40 mL. If resting cardiac index is 2 L/min/m,[2] resting cardiac output for the average man is about 4 L/min. At a heart rate of 70 min, this translates to a forward stroke volume of 57 mL. With a regurgitant volume of 40 mL, the total stroke volume is almost 100 mL. To achieve an ejection fraction of 50%, the end diastolic volume has to be 200 mL. This is about double the normal size, while if there is no MR, the end-diastolic volume would be 114 mL or about normal. Other investigators have also found the negative impact of IMR on survival after myocardial infarction.[10–12]

Some authors argue that IMR is a consequence rather than a cause of postinfarction remodeling[13] and that the impact is in itself not a reason to treat it. Indeed, it is possible that, in some circumstances, the amount of MR is just a marker of the amount of myocardial damage, which is directly related to outcome. However, it has been shown that there is not always a relationship between the amount of myocardial damage on the one hand and occurrence of MR or the grade of MR on the other hand.[10,14] Moreover, it seems unlikely that the damaged ventricle would benefit from MR and not from its abolishment. Theories on the benefit of low afterload for the ventricle in the presence of MR (the pop-off beneficial effect) have no theoretical or practical basis. They probably stem from the observation of bad outcome after mitral valve *replacement* in the presence of severely depressed left ventricular function in the early days of mitral valve surgery.[15]

Given the fact that viable but dysfunctional myocardium can cause IMR explains the observation that after revascularization IMR may resolve. Unfortunately, this is very unpredictable. Christenson[16] argued that mitral valve regurgitation does not need to be treated because in 43 patients with reduced left ventricular (LV)-function, he found that mitral valve regurgitation disappears after revascularization alone.[16] However, only 24 patients had grade II and 7 grade III; 5 patients underwent left ventricular aneurysmectomy, and ejection fraction (EF) improved dramatically (from 18% to 44%) indicating that these patients had severe reversible ischemia and probably little scar. In an elegant observational study, Aklog et al.[17] showed that in patients with pre-operative grade III MR, coronary artery bypass grafting (CABG) alone resolves MR in

only 9% of the cases and 40% persist in grade III or even become grade IV.[17] This was also shown by Czer[18] and Lam.[19] Pre-operative assessment of the segmental viability of the left ventricle might better predict the influence of revascularization alone on IMR, but this strategy is hampered with problems. Viability studies will probably always show some recovery potential in some areas of the ventricle, as this is the indication for the revascularization procedure. Whether the areas that show no reversibility are related to the mechanism of MR will remain unclear. Only when complete reversibility of the ischemia has been predicted, one could hope that IMR resolves after revascularization. Another approach would be to demonstrate the existence of a scar, by using, e.g., late enhancement magnetic resonance imaging (MRI). Unfortunately, the absence of scar tissue does not entirely predict recovery after revascularization. Another problem with both techniques is that even small areas of sustained dysfunction can maintain the MR.[14] Moreover, not only loss of contractility can cause the MR but also dissynchrony can be an important and unpredictable factor after revascularization.[12]

Surgical Treatment of Ischemic Mitral Regurgitation

Considering the above, it makes sense to treat IMR specifically during CABG surgery. The remaining question is however: how can we treat it? Since 2000, we have adopted a strategy of downsizing using a complete semirigid ring with a predefined length of coaptation (at least 8 mm directly after cessation of the extracorporeal circulation (ECC) as end-point (Fig. 10.1c)). In our experience, this can usually be achieved by a 2-size downsizing by means of an Edwards Physio ring, but other rings may need different amounts of downsizing: for instance, the Edwards Classic ring and the St-Jude Medical "saddle shape" ring need only 1-size downsizing to achieve the same result. One should carefully compare the dimensions of the rings. Using this approach in over 100 patients, we found a very low rate of recurrence at follow-up (13% at up to 7 years). Results from several centers have shown disappointing results, especially in the long run. One frequently quoted study, from the Cleveland Clinic group,[20] has especially shown bad results: 6 months after surgery, already 28% had 3+ or 4+ MR. A careful reading of the methods of that paper betrays the use of different rings, no standard sizing, no standard undersizing, no clearly defined end-point at the end of surgery, except the absence of MR, and incomplete follow-up. Most notably, at discharge, already 13% of patients showed recurrence of severe MR. Consequently, the same group[21] tried to dissuade the surgeons from performing an annuloplasty alone in addition to CABG in the presence of severe IMR irrespective of the LV function. Considering the fact that none of our own patients had even a trace of MR at discharge, it is likely that the applied technique is crucial to achieve good late results[22-24]. In many papers that show a high recurrence rate at late follow-up, there is already a considerable recurrence rate at discharge, implying that insufficient or inconsistent downsizing was applied.[25] The reluctance to downsize the mitral annulus is understandable, but our results show low gradients in all fully revalidated patients over a 4-year follow-up[26] while the average coaptation length remains 8 mm. Although the indication for restrictive mitral annuloplasty is grade III or IV MR, due to the dynamic nature of IMR, in patients with grade II MR, an intra-operative loading-test can be performed to assess whether this MR is stable or not.[27]

Another concern might be an unnecessary shrinking of the anterior annulus after downsizing by means of a complete semirigid ring. But in IMR, the mitral annulus loses its shape and becomes flat, which enlarges the anterior intertrigonal distance. By using a saddle-shaped complete rigid or semirigid ring, one may restore the correct length and shape of the anterior annulus.

loplasty; for instance chordal cutting. After first showing experimental benefit of cutting the secondary cords of the anterior mitral valve leaflet[33], Borger also showed clinical benefit in terms of less recurrence of MR.[34] In this study, however, the ring annuloplasty was performed with a partial flexible band, which was only moderately undersized in relationship to the patient's body size, a technique that does not guarantee good results in the first place.[30] Also, it does not seem logical to injure the continuity between mitral valve and left ventricle in already damaged ventricles.

Another addition to annuloplasty is the edge-to-edge technique described by Alfieri[35] (see Chap. 8). In this paper, the authors argue that if coaptation depth is more than 10 mm, annuloplasty does not suffice to create a durable result but that adding an edge-to-edge technique improves results. In our experience, even in patients with severe restriction, downsizing annuloplasty alone will invariably give a good result.[26]

Papillary muscle approximation is another surgical technique to increase leaflet coaptation; its experience is, however, limited to a few clinical reports[36-38] and experimental data.[39] Another adjunct to ring annuloplasty that has been advocated is posterior mitral valve leaflet extension.[40] So far, experimental data show proof of concept but its clinical role remains to be defined.

The Coapsys system is a true alternative to ring annuloplasty: it consists of two epicardially mounted pads connected by a cord that externally compresses the mitral annulus. In a clinical study comparing the Coapsys system with restrictive annuloplasty, the short-term efficacy was shown.[41] Longer studies are needed to clarify its role in the treatment of IMR.

Alternative Surgical Strategies

Besides restrictive annuloplasty, other surgical techniques have been proposed. Obviously, mitral valve replacement with preservation of the subvalvular apparatus is the most dominant alternative. Although some authors showed similar results for repair and replacement[28,29] or in subgroups,[30,31] most studies have shown a clear benefit of repair.[32] Besides, most of the authors then recommend mitral valve replacement using a bioprosthesis; leaving questions about durability. Other techniques are adjunctive procedures to a ring annu-

Outcome of Surgical Treatment

Although we were able to treat IMR with a low recurrence rate, the clinical outcome and ventricular remodeling was varying. In patients with moderately dilated LV (left ventricular end-diastolic volume [LVEDD] <65 mm), 74% showed reverse remodeling, defined as a decrease in LVEDD of 10% compared to pre-op values. However, in patients with severely dilated ventricles (LVEDD >65 mm), only 25% showed reverse remodeling. This lack of reverse remodeling was reflected by the clinical outcome: 5-year survival in the

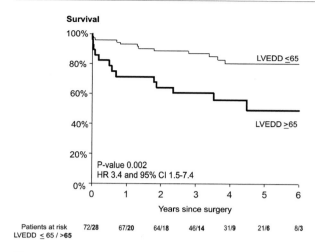

Fig. 10.3 Actuarial survival in 100 patients IMR after restrictive mitral annuloplasty according to the preoperative left ventricular end-diastolic volume (LVEDD) above or below 65 mm (hazard ratio 3.4; 95% confidence interval 1.5–7.4; $p = 0.002$). With permission from Braun et al.[26]

moderately dilated group was 85%, while in the severely dilated group only 40% (Fig. 10.3). Uni- and multivariable analysis showed pre-op LVEDD as the main predictor of outcome and reverse remodeling. Surprisingly, recurrence of MR was not always related to the lack of reverse remodeling: in both groups, about 13% at 4 years.[26]

These results can be interpreted as follows. If ventricular dilatation is limited, surgical treatment of MR (by restrictive annuloplasty) and revascularization is an adequate strategy to improve ventricular function and achieve good late outcome. If, on the other hand, ventricular dilatation has progressed beyond LVEDD >65 mm, this strategy is not sufficient and additional treatments should be considered. This has been the strategy for the last few years in Leiden. Additional treatment depends on the extent of LV dilatation. As long as the LVEDD is between 65 and 80 mm, reconstructing the left ventricle can restore size and shape and therefore function. If the LV has a large postinfarct scar, reshaping the ventricle as in surgical ventricular restoration surgery[42,43] (SVR) yields good results. In patients with more diffuse enlargement of the LV, an external constraint device can limit further dilatation and even reverse it.[44] If LVEDD exceeds 80 mm, reversal of LV function is very unlikely and heart transplantation should be considered. Another option for the extremely enlarged hearts could be a linear plication of

the anterior or lateral wall, as described by Suma et al.[45] Although there is limited experience with this procedure, it needs further research, as most patients in this category are not candidates for transplantation. This above-described approach, CABG, in combination with restrictive mitral annuloplasty (RMA) as the basic strategy and adding LV-procedures depending on LV dilatation, needs further analysis and refining.

An important objection against the treatment of ischemic MR with RMA is that it increases operative risk.[46] In that study, there was a 10% early mortality difference between patients treated with CABG alone or with CABG + RMA. Interestingly, late mortality (at 6 years) was 0 in the repair group and 10% in the CABG only group and suggests that treating IMR – at least in the long run – benefits patients. In most series, no increase in operative risk was found when RMA was added to the procedure.[47] Care should be taken when analyzing the results of patients with IMR operated with CABG only versus CABG + RMA. CABG only patients have, not rarely, less operative risk, since few surgeons are reluctant to leave severe MR untreated, and therefore, selection bias is easily created.

The final issue in the discussion on treatment options for patients with IMR is whether the addition of RMA improves outcome. Although several authors have shown good results in terms of early mortality, early and late absence of MR, reverse remodeling of the left ventricle, no study has yet shown an improvement in survival in a head-to-head comparison study. Despite the need for such a randomized trial, there are arguments that surgically treating IMR indeed improves survival. If we consider our own data, they show a 5-year survival rate of 85% in patients with preoperative LVEDD of less than 65 mm, which seems much better than expected. From a theoretical standpoint, the fact that the left ventricle becomes smaller would infer a survival benefit. Many studies show a relationship of the reverse: as the left ventricle becomes larger, survival becomes less.[48,49] Late survival in patients with more advanced dilatation of the left ventricle is obviously less. But still in these patients, survival is 40% at 5 years, considerably more than in some heart failure trials.[50] Moreover, although we did not see reverse remodeling in these larger ventricles, they also showed little enlargement over time, suggesting stabilization of the disease. In the treatment of heart failure, this would be an important achievement.

In summary, IMR is a disease in itself with a particularly bad prognosis. The surgical treatment is straightforward and consists of a restrictive mitral annuloplasty to achieve an adequate length of coaptation. Good late results, with good survival, good clinical status, and low recurrence rates can be achieved if the end-point of the procedure is not just the mere absence of MR but also the assessment of adequate coaptation of the mitral valve leaflets. Further studies are needed to define the precise survival benefit and to delineate the additional strategies for patients with more extensive disease.

References

1. Ypenburg C, Lancellotti P, Tops LF, et al. Acute effects of initiation and withdrawal of cardiac resynchronization therapy on papillary muscle dyssynchrony and mitral regurgitation. *J Am Coll Cardiol.* 2007;50(21):2071-2077.
2. Ypenburg C, Lancellotti P, Tops LF, et al. Mechanism of improvement in mitral regurgitation after cardiac resynchronization therapy. *Eur Heart J.* 2008;29(6):757-765.
3. Miller GE Jr, Kerth WJ, Gerbode F. Experimental papillary muscle infarction. *J Thorac Cardiovasc Surg.* 1968;56(5):611-616.
4. Gorman RC, McCaughan JS, Ratcliffe MB, et al. Pathogenesis of acute ischemic mitral regurgitation in three dimensions. *J Thorac Cardiovasc Surg.* 1995;109(4):684-693.
5. Komeda M, Glasson JR, Bolger AF, et al. Geometric determinants of ischemic mitral regurgitation. *Circulation.* 1997;96(9 Suppl):II-128-II-133.
6. Kaul S, Spotnitz WD, Glasheen WP. Mechanism of ischemic mitral regurgitation. An experimental evaluation. *Circulation.* 1991;84(5):2167-2180.
7. Grigioni F, Detaint D, Avierinos JF, et al. Contribution of ischemic mitral regurgitation to congestive heart failure after myocardial infarction. *J Am Coll Cardiol.* 2005;45(2):260-267.
8. Grigioni F, Enriquez-Sarano M, Zehr KJ, et al. Ischemic mitral regurgitation: long-term outcome and prognostic implications with quantitative Doppler assessment. *Circulation.* 2001;103(13):1759-1764.
9. Lancellotti P, Gerard PL, Pierard LA. Long-term outcome of patients with heart failure and dynamic functional mitral regurgitation. *Eur Heart J.* 2005;26(15):1528-1532.
10. Lamas GA, Mitchell GF, Flaker GC, et al. Clinical significance of mitral regurgitation after acute myocardial infarction. Survival and Ventricular Enlargement Investigators. *Circulation.* 1997;96(3):827-833.
11. Lehmann KG, Francis CK, Dodge HT. Mitral regurgitation in early myocardial infarction. Incidence, clinical detection, and prognostic implications. TIMI Study Group. *Ann Intern Med.* 1992;117(1):10-17.
12. Trichon BH, Felker GM, Shaw LK, et al. Relation of frequency and severity of mitral regurgitation to survival among patients with left ventricular systolic dysfunction and heart failure. *Am J Cardiol.* 2003;91(5):538-543.
13. Guy TSt, Moainie SL, Gorman JH 3rd, et al. Prevention of ischemic mitral regurgitation does not influence the outcome of remodeling after posterolateral myocardial infarction. *J Am Coll Cardiol.* 2004;43(3):377-383.
14. Frater RW. Ischemic mitral regurgitation. *J Heart Valve Dis.* 1993;2(6):706.
15. Bolling SF, Deeb GM, Brunsting LA, et al. Early outcome of mitral valve reconstruction in patients with end-stage cardiomyopathy. *J Thorac Cardiovasc Surg.* 1995;109(4):676-682. discussion 682–673.
16. Christenson JT, Simonet F, Bloch A, et al. Should a mild to moderate ischemic mitral valve regurgitation in patients with poor left ventricular function be repaired or not? *J Heart Valve Dis.* 1995;4(5):484-488. discussion 488–489.
17. Aklog L, Filsoufi F, Flores KQ, et al. Does coronary artery bypass grafting alone correct moderate ischemic mitral regurgitation? *Circulation.* 2001;104(12 Suppl 1):I68-I75.
18. Czer LS, Maurer G, Bolger AF, et al. Revascularization alone or combined with suture annuloplasty for ischemic mitral regurgitation. Evaluation by color Doppler echocardiography. *Tex Heart Inst J.* 1996;23(4):270-278.
19. Lam BK, Gillinov AM, Blackstone EH, et al. Importance of moderate ischemic mitral regurgitation. *Ann Thorac Surg.* 2005;79(2):462-470. discussion 462–470.
20. McGee EC, Gillinov AM, Blackstone EH, et al. Recurrent mitral regurgitation after annuloplasty for functional ischemic mitral regurgitation. *J Thorac Cardiovasc Surg.* 2004;128(6):916-924.
21. Mihaljevic T, Lam BK, Rajeswaran J, et al. Impact of mitral valve annuloplasty combined with revascularization in patients with functional ischemic mitral regurgitation. *J Am Coll Cardiol.* 2007;49(22):2191-2201.
22. Geidel S, Lass M, Schneider C, et al. Downsizing of the mitral valve and coronary revascularization in severe ischemic mitral regurgitation results in reverse left ventricular and left atrial remodeling. *Eur J Cardiothorac Surg.* 2005;27(6):1011-1016.
23. Geidel S, Schneider C, Lass M, et al. Changes of myocardial function after combined coronary revascularization and mitral valve downsizing in patients with ischemic mitral regurgitation and advanced cardiomyopathy. *Thorac Cardiovasc Surg.* 2007;55(1):1-6.
24. Gelsomino S, Lorusso R, Capecchi I, et al. Left ventricular reverse remodeling after undersized mitral ring annuloplasty in patients with ischemic regurgitation. *Ann Thorac Surg.* 2008;85(4):1319-1330.
25. Serri K, Bouchard D, Demers P, et al. Is a good perioperative echocardiographic result predictive of durability in ischemic mitral valve repair? *J Thorac Cardiovasc Surg.* 2006;131(3):565-573. e562.
26. Braun J, van de Veire NR, Klautz RJ, et al. Restrictive mitral annuloplasty cures ischemic mitral regurgitation and heart failure. *Ann Thorac Surg.* 2008;85(2):430-436. discussion 436–437.
27. Dion R, Benetis R, Elias B, et al. Mitral valve procedures in ischemic regurgitation. *J Heart Valve Dis.* 1995;4(Suppl 2):S124-S129. discussion S129–131.

28. Prifti E, Bonacchi M, Frati G, et al. Ischemic mitral valve regurgitation grade II-III: correction in patients with impaired left ventricular function undergoing simultaneous coronary revascularization. *J Heart Valve Dis.* 2001;10(6):754-762.

29. Prifti E, Bonacchi M, Frati G, et al. Should mild-to-moderate and moderate ischemic mitral regurgitation be corrected in patients with impaired left ventricular function undergoing simultaneous coronary revascularization? *J Card Surg.* 2001;16(6):473-483.

30. Gillinov AM, Wierup PN, Blackstone EH, et al. Is repair preferable to replacement for ischemic mitral regurgitation? *J Thorac Cardiovasc Surg.* 2001;122(6):1125-1141.

31. Calafiore AM, Di Mauro M, Gallina S, et al. Mitral valve surgery for chronic ischemic mitral regurgitation. *Ann Thorac Surg.* 2004;77(6):1989-1997.

32. Akins CW, Hilgenberg AD, Buckley MJ, et al. Mitral valve reconstruction versus replacement for degenerative or ischemic mitral regurgitation. *Ann Thorac Surg.* 1994;58(3):668-675. discussion 675–666.

33. Messas E, Guerrero JL, Handschumacher MD, et al. Chordal cutting: a new therapeutic approach for ischemic mitral regurgitation. *Circulation.* 2001;104(16):1958-1963.

34. Borger MA, Murphy PM, Alam A, et al. Initial results of the chordal-cutting operation for ischemic mitral regurgitation. *J Thorac Cardiovasc Surg.* 2007;133(6):1483-1492.

35. Alfieri O, De Bonis M, Lapenna E, et al. "Edge-to-edge" repair for anterior mitral leaflet prolapse. *Semin Thorac Cardiovasc Surg.* 2004;16(2):182-187.

36. Ueno T, Sakata R, Iguro Y, et al. New surgical approach to reduce tethering in ischemic mitral regurgitation by relocation of separate heads of the posterior papillary muscle. *Ann Thorac Surg.* 2006;81(6):2324-2325.

37. Langer F, Schäfers HJ. RING plus STRING: papillary muscle repositioning as an adjunctive repair technique for ischemic mitral regurgitation. *J Thorac Cardiovasc Surg.* 2007;133(1):247-249.

38. Rama A, Praschker L, Barreda E, et al. Papillary muscle approximation for functional ischemic mitral regurgitation. *Ann Thorac Surg.* 2007;84(6):2130-2131.

39. Hung J, Chaput M, Guerrero JL, et al. Persistent reduction of ischemic mitral regurgitation by papillary muscle repositioning: structural stabilization of the papillary muscle-ventricular wall complex. *Circulation.* 2007;116(11 Suppl):I259-I263.

40. Langer F, Rodriguez F, Cheng A, et al. Posterior mitral leaflet extension: an adjunctive repair option for ischemic mitral regurgitation? *J Thorac Cardiovasc Surg.* 2006;131(4):868-877.

41. Grossi EA, Woo YJ, Schwartz CF, et al. Comparison of Coapsys annuloplasty and internal reduction mitral annuloplasty in the randomized treatment of functional ischemic mitral regurgitation: impact on the left ventricle. *J Thorac Cardiovasc Surg.* 2006;131(5):1095-1098.

42. Di Donato M, Sabatier M, Dor V, et al. Akinetic versus dyskinetic postinfarction scar: relation to surgical outcome in patients undergoing endoventricular circular patch plasty repair. *J Am Coll Cardiol.* 1997;29(7):1569-1575.

43. Menicanti L, Castelvecchio S, Ranucci M, et al. Surgical therapy for ischemic heart failure: single-center experience with surgical anterior ventricular restoration. *J Thorac Cardiovasc Surg.* 2007;134(2):433-441.

44. Starling RC, Jessup M, Oh JK, et al. Sustained benefits of the CorCap Cardiac Support Device on left ventricular remodeling: three year follow-up results from the Acorn clinical trial. *Ann Thorac Surg.* 2007;84(4):1236-1242.

45. Suma H, Tanabe H, Uejima T, et al. Selected ventriculoplasty for idiopathic dilated cardiomyopathy with advanced congestive heart failure: midterm results and risk analysis. *Eur J Cardiothorac Surg.* 2007;32(6):912-916.

46. Kang DH, Kim MJ, Kang SJ, et al. Mitral valve repair versus revascularization alone in the treatment of ischemic mitral regurgitation. *Circulation.* 2006;114(1 Suppl):I499-I503.

47. Diodato MD, Moon MR, Pasque MK, et al. Repair of ischemic mitral regurgitation does not increase mortality or improve long-term survival in patients undergoing coronary artery revascularization: a propensity analysis. *Ann Thorac Surg.* 2004;78(3):794-799. discussion 794–799.

48. Grayburn PA, Appleton CP, DeMaria AN, et al. Echocardiographic predictors of morbidity and mortality in patients with advanced heart failure: the Beta-blocker Evaluation of Survival Trial (BEST). *J Am Coll Cardiol.* 2005;45(7):1064-1071.

49. Hinderliter AL, Blumenthal JA, O'Conner C, et al. Independent prognostic value of echocardiography and N-terminal pro-B-type natriuretic peptide in patients with heart failure. *Am Heart J.* 2008;156(6):1191-1195.

50. St John Sutton M, Pfeffer MA, Moye L, et al. Cardiovascular death and left ventricular remodeling two years after myocardial infarction: baseline predictors and impact of long-term use of captopril: information from the Survival and Ventricular Enlargement (SAVE) trial. *Circulation.* 1997;96(10):3294-3299.

Minimally Invasive Mitral Valve Surgery

11

A. Marc Gillinov and Tomislav Mihaljevic

Introduction

Approaches and techniques for mitral valve surgery are changing, with increasing application of minimally invasive surgical approaches and development of simplified techniques to facilitate repair. Spurred by new technology and instrumentation, increased patient demand, and incipient competition from percutaneous techniques, cardiac surgeons are exhibiting renewed interest in minimally invasive approaches for mitral valve surgery.[1-4] This enthusiasm for minimally invasive mitral valve surgery has been complemented by recent development of simplified techniques for valve repair that reduce operative complexity and time.[5-8] This report will (1) illustrate key technical aspects of the most widely applied minimally invasive approaches for mitral valve surgery, (2) critically examine results of these minimally invasive mitral valve operations in order to determine their safety and effectiveness, and (3) describe recent simplifications in techniques for mitral valve repair that facilitate minimally invasive approaches.

Minimally Invasive Surgical Approaches

In mitral valve surgery, a minimally invasive surgical approach is defined as an operation utilizing a chest wall incision other than median sternotomy.[1-3] The most commonly employed approaches include right

mini-thoracotomy, robotically assisted right thoracic incisions, and partial sternotomy (Fig. 11.1). All provide access to the mitral valve, but they are distinguished by differences in patient preparation, cannulation, and instrumentation.

Right Mini-Thoracotomy

The right mini-thoracotomy approach is increasingly popular for treatment of patients with mitral valve dysfunction and can be employed in those requiring concomitant management of atrial fibrillation or tricuspid regurgitation, as well. Many patients prefer to avoid a sternal incision and therefore request this approach. While minor variations abound, the most common procedure includes a 4–8 cm skin incision in the inframammary crease lateral to the nipple and entry into the chest in the fourth intercostal space[9-14] (Fig. 11.1). Patient preparation includes a double lumen endotracheal tube and positioning with a roll under the right scapula; the right arm is distracted 5–10 cm to provide working room for the surgeon and to enable placement of a transthoracic clamp (Fig. 11.2). After entry into the fourth intercostal space, a soft tissue retractor is placed to improve exposure and to protect the intercostal neurovascular bundle. The standard stainless steel rib retractor is positioned next. Occasionally, the diaphragm obscures exposure of the pericardium near the inferior vena cava; a stay suture in the diaphragm, brought out through the fifth or sixth intercostal space, can improve exposure. The pericardium is opened 3 cm or more anterior to the phrenic nerve and stay sutures brought through the chest wall in the mid-axillary line retract the pericardium. While some surgeons employ videoscopic techniques, the procedure is easily performed under direct visualization.

A.M. Gillinov (✉)
Atrial Fibrillation Center, Department of Thoracic and Cardiovascular Surgery, Cleveland Clinic Foundation, Cleveland, Ohio
e-mail: gillinom@ccf.org

R.S. Bonser et al. (eds.), *Mitral Valve Surgery*,
DOI: 10.1007/978-1-84996-426-5_11, © Springer-Verlag London Limited 2011

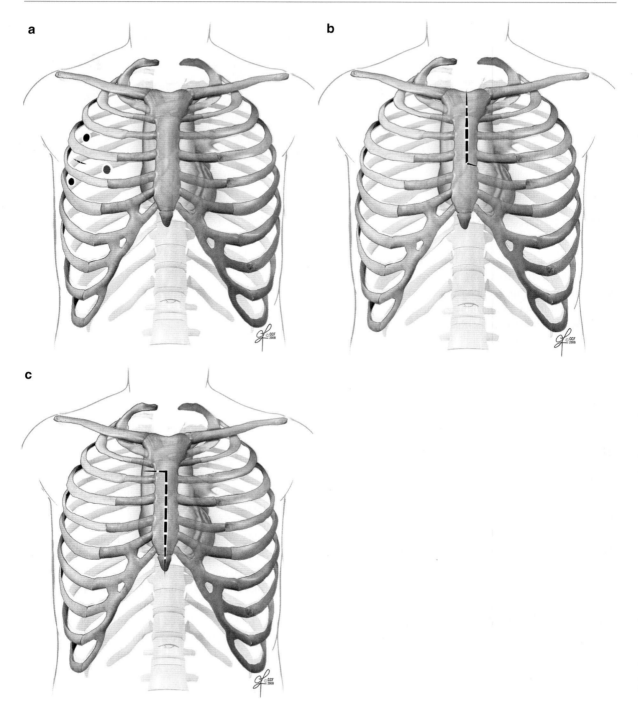

Fig. 11.1 Minimally invasive approaches for mitral valve surgery. (**a**) robotically assisted right-sided approach demonstrating working port (fourth intercostal space, lateral), left arm port (third intercostal space), right arm port (fifth intercostal space), and camera port (fourth intercostal space, medial). A separate port for a dynamic left atrial retractor may be placed in the fourth or fifth intercostal space. Port placement varies based on body habitus; (**b**) partial upper sternotomy; (**c**) partial lower sternotomy (Reprinted with permission, Cleveland Clinic Center for Medical Art & Photography © 2006–2010. All Rights Reserved)

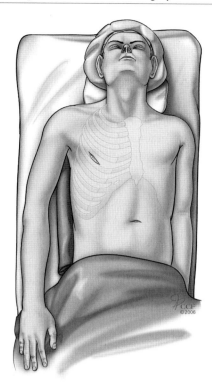

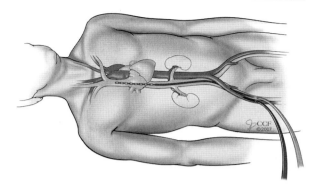

Fig. 11.3 Right mini-thoracotomy: Cannulation. The femoral venous cannula is advanced into the superior vena cava using guidewire technique and echo guidance (Reprinted with permission, Cleveland Clinic Center for Medical Art & Photography © 2006–2010. All Rights Reserved)

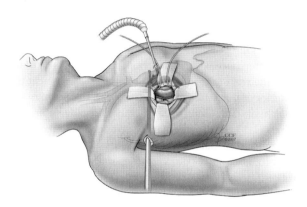

Fig. 11.2 Right mini-thoracotomy: Patient preparation. The right arm is distracted from the torso to facilitate placement of a transthoracic aortic cross-clamp (Reprinted with permission, Cleveland Clinic Center for Medical Art & Photography © 2006–2010. All Rights Reserved)

Fig. 11.4 Right mini-thoracotomy: Cardioplegia and mitral valve exposure. A transthoracic clamp is depicted entering the chest in the third interspace. Antegrade and retrograde cardioplegia are employed. A static atrial retractor aids in valve exposure (Reprinted with permission, Cleveland Clinic Center for Medical Art & Photography © 2006–2010. All Rights Reserved)

Cardiopulmonary bypass is established by peripheral cannulation (Fig. 11.3). The anterior surfaces of the femoral artery and vein are exposed and cannulated with Seldinger technique. Under echo guidance, the venous cannula is advanced into the superior vena cava; the leading edge of the cannula should be at least 4 cm into the superior vena cava to prevent migration back into the right atrium, which can cause inadequate drainage and obscure exposure of the mitral valve. If the patient is very large or if drainage is inadequate, a second venous cannula is placed in the superior vena cava either directly through the incision or percutaneously via the right internal jugular vein. Aortic occlusion is accomplished with a transthoracic clamp inserted through the third intercostal space in the midaxillary line; alternative methods of aortic occlusion include a flexible clamp introduced into the field, or an endoaortic balloon introduced via the femoral arterial cannula and positioned with echo guidance. We favor the transthoracic clamp when using the nonrobotic right mini-thoracotomy approach.[15] Myocardial protection is achieved with antegrade cardioplegia (catheter placed directly in ascending aorta or endoaortic balloon) and is frequently supplemented by retrograde cardioplegia and systemic cooling (Fig. 11.4). Some surgeons prefer to perform the valve procedure on the fibrillating heart and do not occlude the aorta or employ cardioplegia; this approach generally entails systemic cooling to 20–25°C.

The mitral valve is approached via a standard left atriotomy. A static retractor placed through the third intercostal space lateral to the internal thoracic artery retracts the interatrial septum and exposes the mitral valve. Long-shafted instruments are used to perform the repair. Placement of annuloplasty sutures before leaflet repair improves exposure, particularly in the region of P3. A knot-pusher is used to tie sutures, as tying by hand is not possible with this approach.

Robotically Assisted Right Thoracic Approach

Robotically assisted mitral valve repair entails a right thoracic approach.[16–20] Mastery of standard, minimally invasive, nonrobotic right thoracotomy technique is mandatory before progressing to robotically assisted surgery. The robotic, port-based approach includes a working port in the fourth intercostal space anterior to the anterior axillary line and a camera port in the fourth intercostal space two to three fingerbreadths anterior to the working port. The left robotic arm is placed in the third interspace 3–5 cm anterior to the anterior axillary line, the right arm in the fifth or sixth interspace at the anterior axillary line, and the atrial retractor arm in the fourth or fifth interspace in the mid-clavicular line (Fig. 11.1). Port placement is crucial and may vary depending on patient body habitus. It is particularly important to have sufficient separation between the robotic arms in order to avoid instrument conflicts. Cardiopulmonary bypass is established after cannulation of the femoral artery and vein, and venous drainage is frequently augmented by a cannula in the superior vena cava introduced via the right internal jugular vein. As with a standard thoracotomy approach, aortic occlusion is achieved with a transthoracic clamp or the endoaortic balloon; the endoaortic balloon is preferred in patients with normal dimension of the ascending aorta (less than 3.7 cm in diameter). Myocardial protection may include antegrade cardioplegia, retrograde cardioplegia (via a percutaneous coronary sinus catheter), and moderate systemic hypothermia (cooling to 30°C).

Partial Sternotomy

While there was great initial enthusiasm for the partial sternotomy approach to mitral valve repair, this has recently been supplanted by interest in right-sided incisions that do not involve division of the sternum.

The mitral valve can be approached via a 6–8 cm midline skin incision followed by either upper or lower partial sternotomy[21–23] (Fig. 11.1). With both approaches, central arterial cannulation and direct aortic cross-clamping are employed, making this the minimally invasive approach of choice in patients with small femoral arteries or peripheral arterial disease. With an upper sternotomy, venous drainage is achieved via separate cannulation of the superior and inferior vena cavae, while femoral venous cannulation is used with a partial lower sternotomy. Antegrade cardioplegia is delivered via a catheter placed directly in the ascending aorta. Mitral valve exposure with partial upper sternotomy is obtained through an extended transseptal incision. When partial lower sternotomy is used, the mitral valve can be exposed via standard left atriotomy or via a transseptal approach. With a partial sternotomy approach, standard instrumentation is used for the repair, and sutures are tied by hand.

Minimally Invasive Approaches: Comparison of Technical Considerations and Patient Selection

Each of the three approaches places distinct requirements on the surgical team for preparation of the patient and execution of the operative plan (Table 11.1). While partial sternotomy does not require additional nonstandard maneuvers by the anesthesiologist, right thoracic approaches are facilitated by a double lumen endotracheal tube. Robotically assisted surgery requires bilateral blood pressure monitoring if an endoaortic balloon is employed for aortic occlusion; in addition, it is advantageous to have the ability to deliver retrograde cardioplegia via a coronary sinus catheter placed by the anesthesiologist. Surgical instrumentation is standard with a partial sternotomy, and the learning curve is short. In contrast, specially designed long-shafted instruments are employed with right thoracic approaches. Of course, preprocedure familiarization with the surgical robot is mandatory before performing robotically assisted surgery.

Patient selection influences the choice of surgical approach. While there are few absolute contraindications, we believe that there are several relative contraindications to right thoracic approaches (Table 11.2).

Table 11.1 Minimally invasive approaches: technical considerations

	Partial sternotomy	Right mini-thoracotomy	Robotically assisted
Anesthesia preparation	Standard	Double lumen ETT	Double lumen ETT Bilateral art lines Retrograde cardioplegia catheter
Cannulation	Central	Peripheral	Peripheral
Myocardial protection	Antegrade/retrograde	Antegrade/retrograde Systemic hypothermia[a]	Antegrade/retrograde Systemic hypothermia[b]
Instrumentation	Standard	Long-shafted	Robotic
Visualization	Good	Good	Excellent
Learning curve	5 cases	10 cases	20 cases
Cross-clamp time	45–75 min	45–75 min	60–120 min

ETT, endotracheal tube; art, arterial
[a]Systemic hypothermia may be used without cardioplegia
[b]Systemic hypothermia is used as an adjunct to cardioplegia

Table 11.2 Minimally invasive approaches: relative contraindications

	Partial sternotomy	Right mini-thoracotomy	Robotically assisted
Annular calcification	No[a]	Yes	Yes
Descending aortic atherosclerosis	No	Yes[b]	Yes
Peripheral arterial disease	No	Yes	Yes
Aortic regurgitation (>1+)	No	Yes	Yes
Small femoral artery	No	Yes	Yes
Mitral replacement	No	No	Yes

[a]Full sternotomy is advisable in the setting of severe mitral annular calcification
[b]In the setting of severe ascending aortic atherosclerosis, some favor peripheral cannulation and a right thoracotomy approach to the mitral valve

When such contraindications exist, we favor a partial sternotomy for minimally invasive mitral valve surgery.

Results of Minimally Invasive Mitral Valve Surgery

Valve Repair

The literature is filled with reports of single center and multicenter experiences documenting results of minimally invasive mitral valve surgery.

It is clear that the mitral valve can be repaired or replaced via partial sternotomy, right thoracotomy, or a port-based robotically assisted approach.[1] With an experienced team, the probability of repair is not diminished by a minimally invasive approach.[23–28] In fact, some suggest that superior visualization and exposure associated with robotically assisted surgery might increase repair rates.[18] Need for conversion to sternotomy ranges from 0% to 5% with minimally invasive approaches, with no particular approach being substantially less likely to require conversion.

Mortality and Morbidity

In appropriately selected patients, minimally invasive approaches do not increase hospital mortality. However, minimally invasive approaches invite certain complications that are less common with sternotomy. Peripheral cannulation, which is used with right thoracic approaches, is associated with a 1% risk of peripheral vascular complications; although rare, aortic dissection is a potentially life-threatening complication of femoral artery instrumentation and perfusion.[29] The endoaortic balloon adds cost and complexity and requires special training. Its deployment has been associated with aortic dissection, inadequate myocardial protection, and damage to the aortic valve[24,25,29,30]; however, these adverse events are very uncommon in experienced hands. Robotic procedures are universally associated with longer cross-clamp times than are other approaches, and this may result in increased inotrope requirements in the early perioperative period.[18] Recognizing this, we employ antegrade and retrograde cardioplegia and moderate systemic hypothermia (30°C) during robotically assisted mitral valve surgery. With experience and application of simplified repair techniques (see later), operative times for robotically assisted procedures can be decreased substantially.

Partial sternotomy approaches include central arterial cannulation and standard techniques for cardioplegia delivery. These features simplify the procedure and reduce the risk of peripheral vascular complications. Partial upper sternotomy is a versatile approach, which allows unrestricted access to the entire ascending aorta and the aortic, mitral, and tricuspid valves; it is therefore a good choice for patients with multivalvular disease. However, the use of an extended transseptal incision with partial upper sternotomy increases the incidence of postoperative bradyarrhythmias. A lower hemi-sternotomy occasionally results in inadequate mitral valve exposure, requiring low-risk conversion to full sternotomy.[31] After completing the learning curve, mitral valve repair via partial sternotomy does not take longer than repair via full sternotomy.[21–23]

Benefits of Minimally Invasive Mitral Valve Surgery

Proposed benefits of minimally invasive mitral valve surgery include improved cosmesis, shorter hospital length of stay, faster return to normal activity, lower transfusion requirement, cost savings, reduced postoperative pain, lower risk of wound infection, and fewer pulmonary complications.[1] The magnitude of these benefits may vary with the particular minimally invasive approach employed (Table 11.3).

Cosmesis

With a smaller incision than standard median sternotomy, each of the minimally invasive approaches is clearly associated with improved cosmesis. This is important to many patients. In a study of patients having right thoracotomy, Casselman and colleagues found that 99% of patients felt that their scar was aesthetically pleasing.[13] Which procedure results in the

Table 11.3 Minimally invasive approaches: outcome comparisons

	Partial sternotomy	Right mini-thoracotomy	Robotically assisted
Cosmesis	++	+++	++++
Postoperative pain	++	++	+++
Postoperative NSR	++	+++	+++
Short ICU length of stay	+++	++++	++++
Short hospital length of stay	+++	++++	++++
Transfusion requirement	+++	+++	++++
Wound infection	++	+++	++++
Cost	++++	+++	++

NSR, normal sinus rhythm; ICU, intensive care unit
++ Good
+++ Very good
++++ Excellent

best cosmesis is a matter of contention. Many patients prefer not to have a midline incision or any sort of sternotomy, and this may be responsible for the proliferation of programs offering right thoracic approaches. Improved cosmesis is the only undisputed benefit of minimally invasive surgery.[24]

Postoperative Pain

The small thoracotomy incision used for right thoracic approaches is associated with limited discomfort, and pain is further minimized by avoiding rib-spreading.[13] Compared to patients having sternotomy, those having right mini-thoracotomy have similar pain for the first 2 postoperative days and less pain from postoperative day 3 onward.[32] When compared to full sternotomy, partial sternotomy has been associated with reduced need for postoperative analgesics.[33] Lower narcotic requirements may have the added benefit of reducing the incidence of postoperative delirium.[33] Overall, it does appear that the minimally invasive approaches are associated with less postoperative pain than is standard sternotomy.

Hospital Length of Stay and Recovery

Right thoracotomy approaches are associated with hospital length of stay of 4–6 days, and a case-control study demonstrated that this is generally shorter than the length of stay after sternotomy.[27] However, this finding of reduced length of stay is not supported by all studies.[24] After right mini-thoracotomy, approximately half of the patients return to work and full activity within 4 weeks.[13] After robotic mitral valve repair, length of stay is similarly 4–6 days,[16–20] and comparative studies suggest that this is shorter than that achieved in similar patients undergoing sternotomy.[26,30] However, the length of stay varies with institutional practices and policies, and it is difficult to draw firm conclusions that are generally applicable.[16–20,30] With an aggressive strategy of early discharge, some surgeons have managed to discharge one third of patients within 24 h of robotically assisted surgery; however, nearly half of these patients required hospital readmission.[20] Like right thoracic approaches, partial sternotomy is accompanied by median length of stay of 4–6 days, and when compared to full sternotomy, appears more likely to result in earlier discharge to home.[19–23,34]

Thus, patients do seem to leave the hospital somewhat earlier after minimally invasive mitral valve surgery.

Transfusion

Transfusion requirements depend as much on individual institutional policy as on surgical approach, with 15–74% of patients receiving transfusion in different series of patients having minimally invasive mitral valve surgery. In a case-control study, Grossi and colleagues found that the right thoracotomy approach was associated with fewer transfusions than was the sternotomy approach, but 52% of minimally invasive patients received blood products in this report.[27] Transfusion requirements are low in robotic series, with 20–45% of patients requiring transfusion after robotically assisted mitral valve repair.[17,18,20] After partial sternotomy, approximately 25% of patients require transfusion.[21–23] It is likely that a smaller incision is associated with lower probability of transfusion, but this has not been proven conclusively.

Wound Infection

Infection of right thoracic incisions is extremely rare, and this approach virtually eliminates the occurrence of mediastinitis.[27] In contrast, mediastinitis is uncommon but possible after partial sternotomy.

Cost

Right mini-thoracotomy approaches require special instrumentation and retractors that entail a small, initial capital investment. There are no special additional hospital costs thereafter. In contrast, robotic cardiac surgery is associated with a large initial capital investment, a service contract for the robot, and disposable costs for the robotic arms; in addition, there are expenses related to the endoaortic balloon and the retrograde cardioplegia catheter, if used. However, it has been suggested that reduced hospital length of stay and earlier return to full function offset the increase in total hospital cost for robotically assisted approaches[35]; therefore, robotically assisted surgery may have a broad, positive economic impact. Compared to sternotomy, partial sternotomy has been associated with decreased hospital costs because of earlier hospital discharge.[21–23,34]

Benefits: Summary

There are few comparative data substantiating the wide-ranging medical benefits that have been attributed to minimally invasive surgery.[1] The cosmetic benefit is certain, and there does seem to be reduction in length of stay and lower requirement for blood products. It is not clear that any of the approaches is absolutely superior to the others in terms of clinical outcome. Therefore, choice of procedure depends on patient's desire, patient's characteristics, and surgical expertise.

Repair Techniques

Recent increased interest in minimally invasive approaches to mitral valve surgery has been complemented by introduction (or re-introduction) of surgical techniques that simplify mitral valve repair. These mitral valve repair techniques help to reduce operative time, easing the learning curve associated with minimally invasive approaches. The specific repair technique applied depends primarily on the site of prolapse. All leaflet and chordal repair techniques are accompanied by incorporation of an annuloplasty.

Posterior Prolapse

Approximately 75% of patients with mitral regurgitation caused by degenerative disease have isolated prolapse of the posterior leaflet, most commonly the P2 segment (middle scallop).[36] The classic technique for managing this is quadrangular resection, with or without sliding repair.[37] The sliding repair was developed to reduce the risk of post-repair left ventricular outflow tract obstruction from systolic anterior motion (SAM) of the mitral valve in the setting of excessive leaflet tissue and/or a small, hyperdynamic left ventricle.[38] In our clinical practice, we have replaced standard quadrangular resection and sliding repair with triangular resection and folding plasty, respectively;

these two simplified techniques for correction of posterior leaflet prolapse reduce the number of surgical maneuvers and thereby decrease operative time.

Triangular Resection

In the patient with segmental posterior leaflet prolapse, mitral regurgitation is caused by lack of coaptation at the site of chordal rupture or elongation. Therefore, it is logical to target the prolapsing free edge of the leaflet when addressing this problem. A triangular resection entails resection of the portion of the free edge that prolapses, with incisions in the leaflet angled toward one another as the incision approaches the annular level.[5,6] No annular plication sutures are necessary as in a standard quadrangular resection; this simplifies the procedure and reduces the risk of circumflex artery distortion or kinking.

Folding Plasty

The folding plasty is used to treat posterior leaflet prolapse when there is a high risk of SAM, replacing the sliding repair in such cases.[8] The prolapsing portion of the posterior leaflet is resected as for a quadrangular resection, leaving tall posterior leaflet remnants on either side. These remnants are folded down to the annulus by taking a suture through the mid-portion of each cut edge and passing the suture through the annulus in the region of the resection. This reduces the leaflet height. Leaflet tissue is then approximated to the annulus, closing the gap at the annular level and uniformly reducing the height of the posterior leaflet in this region. The leaflet edges are reapproximated in the middle and an annuloplasty completes the repair.

Anterior Prolapse

Correction of anterior leaflet prolapse is traditionally more challenging than is correction of posterior leaflet prolapse. Classic techniques for management of anterior leaflet prolapse include chordal transfer, which usually requires manipulation of the posterior leaflet, chordal shortening, which is associated with reduced durability, and triangular resection.[39] Management of anterior prolapse by creation of artificial chordae simplifies the procedure.

Artificial chordae are usually constructed of ePTFE (Gore-Tex, W.L. Gore and Assoc, Flagstaff, AZ). The key challenge with the creation of artificial chordae is determination of chordal length, and there are many techniques for estimating the chordal length.[40,41] We favor use of a caliper for direct measurement and construction of chordal loops, as described by Von Uppell and Mohr.[40] With this technique, the caliper is used to measure the length of a normal chord or, if there is no reference chord, the distance from the papillary muscle head to the annulus. Chordal loops of this length are constructed and affixed to a papillary muscle; for repair of anterior prolapse, length is most commonly 22–24 mm. Finally, the loops are affixed to the free edge of the prolapsing leaflet with a Gore-Tex suture. This technique may also be applied for correction of posterior leaflet prolapse.

Commissural Prolapse

Commissuroplasty is a simple and reproducible solution for management of commissural prolapse involving the anterior leaflet, posterior leaflet, or both leaflets.[42] The edge of the prolapsing segment is sutured to the free edge of the opposite leaflet. A relatively large annuloplasty device is employed to avoid mitral stenosis.

Recommendations

When faced with the need for mitral valve surgery, patients tend to focus on (1) valve repair (versus replacement) and (2) minimally invasive approaches. Increasingly, well-informed patients wish to avoid a standard sternotomy. Although excellent results are achieved with sternotomy and there are potential advantages related to de-airing the heart and management of uncommon complications (e.g., intraoperative aortic dissection, coronary artery impingement), patients often prefer less invasive approaches.

Therefore, surgeons experienced in mitral valve repair should develop expertise in one or more minimally invasive approaches in order to meet patients' needs. Application of simplified repair techniques makes minimally invasive mitral valve repair accessible to more surgeons. When choosing a minimally invasive approach in a particular patient, anatomic and pathologic factors must be considered in order to optimize safety and maximize the probability of valve repair. The informed consent process should include discussion of potential limitations and risks associated with each operative approach.

Future Directions

Surgeons must complement application of less invasive chest wall approaches with innovation in technology for mitral valve repair. Devices and instruments that facilitate or replace knot tying have the potential to reduce operative times and lower the barrier to entry for surgeons.[43] When commercially available, annuloplasty rings that incorporate automatic techniques for fixation will become essential components of minimally invasive mitral valve operations. Artificial chordae that are prepackaged and include tissue fixation technology for attachment to the papillary muscle will further simplify repairs. The next advances in minimally invasive mitral valve surgery require development of a suite of repair devices and techniques that minimize traditional "cut-and-sew" surgical technique and facilitate rapid, reliable valve repair through tiny incisions or ports.

References

1. Rosengart TK, Feldman T, Borger MA, et al. Percutaneous and minimally invasive valve procedures: A scientific statement from the American Heart Association council on cardiovascular surgery and anesthesia, council on clinical cardiology, functional genomics, and translation biology interdisciplinary working group, and quality of care and outcomes research interdisciplinary working group. *Circulation.* 2008; 117:1750-1767.
2. Woo YJ, Rodriguez E, Atluri P, Chitwood WR Jr. Minimally invasive, robotic, and off-pump mitral valve surgery. *Semin Thorac Cardiovasc Surg.* 2006;18:139-147.
3. Caffarelli AD, Robbins RC. Will minimally invasive vale replacement ever really be important? *Curr Opin Cardiol.* 2004;19:123-127.

4. AACF, AHA, Vassiliades TA Jr, Block PC, Cohn LH, et al. The clinical development of percutaneous heart valve technology: a position statement of the Society of Thoracic Surgeons (STS), the American Association for Thoracic Surgery (AATS), and the Society for Cardiovascular Angiography and Interventions (SCAI). *J Thorac Cardiovasc Surg.* 2005;129:970–976.

5. Brown ML, Abel MD, Click RL, et al. Systolic anterior motion after mitral valve repair: is surgical intervention necessary? *J Thorac Cardiovasc Surg.* 2007;133:136-143.

6. Da Col U, Di Bella I, Bardelli G, Koukoulis G, Ramoni E, Ragni T. Triangular resection and folding of posterior leaflet for mitral valve repair. *J Card Surg.* 2006;21:274-276.

7. Lapenna E, Torracca L, De Bonis M, La Canna G, Crescenzi G, Alferi O. Minimally invasive mitral valve repair in the context of Barlow's disease. *Ann Thorac Surg.* 2005;79:1496-1499.

8. Calafiore AM, Di Mauro M, Iaco AL, et al. Overreduction of the posterior annulus in surgical treatment of degenerative mitral regurgitation. *Ann Thorac Surg.* 2006;81:1310-1316.

9. Grossi EA, Galloway AC, La Pietra A, et al. Minimally invasive mitral valve surgery: a 6-year experience with 714 patients. *Ann Thorac Surg.* 2002;74:660-664.

10. Aybek T, Dogan S, Risteski PS, et al. Two hundred forty minimally invasive mitral operations through right minithoracotomy. *Ann Thorac Surg.* 2006;81:1618-1624.

11. Glower DD, Siegel LC, Frischmeyer KJ, et al. Predictors of outcome in a multicenter port-access valve registry. *Ann Thorac Surg.* 2000;70:1054-1059.

12. Casselman FP, Van Slycke S, Dom H, Lambrechts DL, Vermeulen Y, Vanermen H. Endoscopic mitral valve repair: feasibility, reproducible, and durable. *J Thorac Cardiovasc Surg.* 2003;125:273-282.

13. Casselman FP, Van Slycke S, Wellens F, et al. Mitral valve surgery can now routinely be performed endoscopically. *Circulation.* 2003;108(suppl II):II-48-II-54.

14. Walther T, Falk V, Mohr FW. Minimally invasive mitral valve surgery. *J Cardiovasc Surg.* 2004;45(5):487-495.

15. Chitwood WR, Elbeery JR, Moran JF, Minimally Invasive Surgery Workgroup. Minimally invasive mitral valve repair using transthoracic aortic occlusion. *Ann Thorac Surg.* 1997;63:1477-1479.

16. Siwek LG, Reynolds B. Totally robotic mitral valve repair. *Op Tech Thorac Cardiovasc Surg.* 2007;12:235-249.

17. Nifong LW, Chitwood WR, Pappas PS, et al. for the Multi-Center Robotic Mitral Repair Group. Robotic mitral valve surgery: a United States multicenter trial. *J Thorac Cardiovasc Surg.* 2005;129:1395–1404.

18. Murphy DA, Miller JS, Langford DA, Snyder AB. Endoscopic robotic mitral valve surgery. *J Thorac Cardiovasc Surg.* 2006;132:776-781.

19. Rodriguez E, Nifong LW, Chu MWA, Wood W, Vos PW, Chitwood WR. Robotic mitral valve repair for anterior leaflet and bileaflet prolapse. *Ann Thorac Surg.* 2008;85:438-444.

20. Tatooles AJ, Pappas PS, Gordon PJ, Slaughter MS. Minimally invasive mitral valve repair using the da Vinci robotic system. *Ann Thorac Surg.* 2004;77:1978-1984.

21. Greelish JP, Cohn LH, Leacche M, et al. Minimally invasive mitral valve repair suggests earlier operation for mitral valve disease. *J Thorac Cardiovasc Surg.* 2003;126:365-373.

22. Gillinov AM, Cosgrove DM. Minimally invasive mitral valve surgery: Mini-sternotomy with extended transseptal approach. *Semin Thorac Cardiovasc Surg.* 1999;3:206-211.

23. Mihaljevic T, Cohn LH, Unic D, Aranki SF, Couper GS, Byrne JG. One thousand minimally invasive valve operations: early and late results. *Ann Surg.* 2004;240:529-534.

24. Dogan S, Aybek T, Risteski PS, et al. Minimally invasive port access versus conventional mitral valve surgery: prospective randomized study. *Ann Thorac Surg.* 2005;79:492-498.

25. Reichenspurner H, Detter C, Deuse T, Boehm DH, Treede H, Reichart B. Video and robotic-assisted minimally invasive mitral valve surgery: A comparison of the port-access and transthoracic clamp techniques. *Ann Thorac Surg.* 2005;79:485-491.

26. Folliguet T, Vanhuyse F, Constantino X, Realli M, Laborde F. Mitral valve repair robotic versus sternotomy. *Eur J Cardiothorac Surg.* 2006;29:362-366.

27. Grossi EA, Galloway AC, Ribakove GH, et al. Impact of minimally invasive valvular heart surgery: a case-control study. *Ann Thorac Surg.* 2001;71:807-810.

28. Grossi EA, La Pietra A, Ribakove GH, et al. Minimally invasive versus sternotomy approaches for mitral reconstruction: Comparison of intermediate-term results. *J Thorac Cardiovasc Surg.* 2001;121:708-713.

29. Jeanmart H, Casselman FP, De Grieck Y, et al. Avoiding vascular complications during minimally invasive, totally endoscopic intracardiac surgery. *J Thorac Cardiovasc Surg.* 2007;133:1066-1070.

30. Woo YJ, Nacke EA. Robotic minimally invasive mitral valve reconstruction yields less blood product transfusion and shorter length of stay. *Surgery.* 2006;140:263-267.

31. Tabata M, Umakanthan R, Khalpey Z, et al. Conversion to full sternotomy during minimal-access cardiac surgery: reasons and results during a 9.5 year experience. *J Thorac Cardiovasc Surg.* 2007;134:165-169.

32. Walther T, Falk V, Metz S, et al. Pain and quality of life after minimally invasive versus conventional cardiac surgery. *Ann Thorac Surg.* 1999;67:1643-1647.

33. Yamada T, Ochiai R, Takeda J, Shin H, Yozu R. Comparison of early postoperative quality of life in minimally invasive versus conventional valve surgery. *J Anesth.* 2003;17:171-176.

34. Cohn LH, Adams DH, Couper GS, et al. Minimally invasive cardiac valve surgery improves patient satisfaction while reducing costs of cardiac valve replacement and repair. *Ann Surg.* 1997;226(4):421-426. discussion 427–428.

35. Morgan JA, Thornton BA, Peacock JC, et al. Does robotic technology make minimally invasive cardiac surgery too expensive? A hospital cost analysis of robotic and conventional techniques. *J Card Surg.* 2005;20:246-251.

36. Gillinov AM, Cosgrove DM, Blackstone EH, et al. Durability of mitral valve repair for degenerative disease. *J Thorac Cardiovasc Surg.* 1998;116:734-743.

37. Braunberger E, Deloche A, Berrebi A, et al. Very long-term results (more than 20 years) of valve repair with Carpentier's techniques in nonrheumatic mitral valve insufficiency. *Circulation.* 2001;104([suppl I]I):I-8-I-11.

38. Cosgrove GAM, III DM. Modified sliding leaflet technique for repair of the mitral valve. *Ann Thorac Surg*. 1999;68: 2356-2357.
39. Gillinov AM, Cosgrove DM III. Chordal transfer for repair of anterior leaflet prolapse. *Semin Thorac Cardiovasc Surg*. 2004;16:169-173.
40. Von Oppel UO, Mohr FW. Chordal replacement for both minimally invasive and conventional mitral valve surgery using premeasured Gore-Tex loops. *Ann Thorac Surg*. 2000; 70:2166-2168.
41. Gillinov AM, Banbury MK. Pre-measured artificial chordae for mitral valve repair. *Ann Thorac Surg*. 2007;84: 2127-2129.
42. Gillinov AM, Shortt KG, Cosgrove DM III. Commissural closure for repair of mitral commissural prolapse. *Ann Thorac Surg*. 2005;80:1135-1136.
43. Cook RC, Nifong LW, Enterkin JE, et al. Significant reduction in annuloplasty operative time with the use of nitinol clips in robotically assisted mitral valve repair. *J Thorac Cardiovasc Surg*. 2007;133:1264-1267.

Mitral Stenosis

Jose Luis Pomar and Daniel Pereda

Etiology and Epidemiology

The main cause of mitral stenosis (MS) continues to be today undoubtedly, as it has been in the past, rheumatic heart disease. Pure MS occurs in about 40% of patients with rheumatic heart disease and about two thirds of them are females. On the other hand, the antecedent of rheumatic fever is encountered on anamnesis in more than 60% of patients presenting with isolated MS.[1,2]

Other much less frequent conditions producing MS are: congenital (usually presenting in the pediatric population), mucopolysaccharidosis, carcinoid tumor (malignant forms), systemic lupus erythematosus, rheumatic arthritis, Whipple disease, Fabry disease, and mitral annular calcification in the elderly. Patients under treatment with methysergide may unusually develop MS. Other entities that may simulate typical MS findings are: left atrial myxomas (must be discarded when first evaluating a patient with probable MS), cor triatriatum, congenital left atrium membranes, and cases of infective endocarditis with large vegetations on the mitral valve.

In patients with prior mitral valve replacement (MVR), prosthesis thrombosis or dysfunction and pannus formation may reproduce the clinical and hemodynamic picture of typical rheumatic MS.

Pathology and Pathophysiology

The typical rheumatic stenotic mitral valve has a funnel shape and a small central orifice with a "fish mouth" configuration accompanied by thickening and fibrosis

J.L. Pomar (✉)
The Thoracic Institute Hospital Clinic,
University of Barcelona, Barcelona, Spain
e-mail: jlpomar@clinic.ub.es

of the leaflets and chordae. Calcium deposits can develop in the injured leaflets (Fig. 12.1). This calcification often extends into the mitral annulus, especially into the posterior segments making the valve even more rigid and complicating the possible repair.

The main features in rheumatic MS are leaflet thickening and their fusion in the commissural area (Fig. 12.2). This thickening of the leaflets is uneven and is usually more evident at their free margin and in the fused areas.

The involvement of the chordae and the rest of the subvalvular apparatus is very variable and there can be a severe obstruction to flow through the valve with nearly normal chords and papillary. However, there usually exist some degree of chordal thickening (Fig. 12.3), fusion, and retraction creating an anatomical spectrum of MS that ranges from the isolated alteration on any of these structures to severe combined destruction of all of them with profuse calcification extending to the annulus and even into the left atrium, left ventricle and papillary muscles. Calcification increases as does the age of the patients, usually beginning in the fused commissures.

Pure MS of clinical significance is normally accompanied by left atrial enlargement and increased wall thickness. Left ventricle is usually normal in size, shape, and function. Patients with profuse annulus calcification may have regional wall motion abnormalities in their basal left ventricle segments.[3]

The normal mitral valve in adults has an opening area during diastole of about 4–6 cm^2 that allows ventricular filling from the left atrium with a gradient that approaches zero. As mitral stenosis develops, this area is gradually and slowly reduced over the years and when it is around 2 cm^2 (mild MS), the left ventricle can only be filled in diastole by means of an abnormally elevated atrioventricular gradient. As valve area further reduces, this

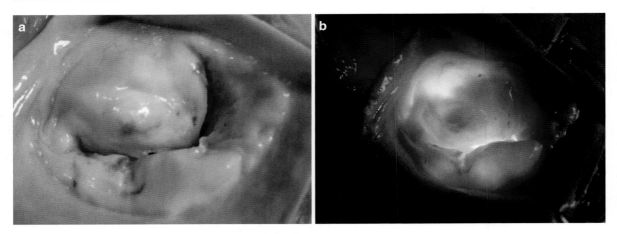

Fig. 12.1 (**a**) Explanted mitral valve showing the typical features of rheumatic mitral stenosis. (**b**) The same specimen has been transilluminated for a better demonstration of the irregular thickening of the leaflets

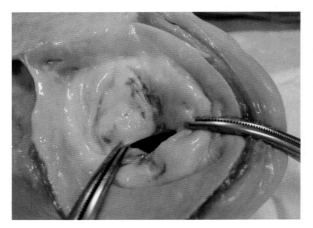

Fig. 12.2 The same valve shown in Fig. 12.1 is examined to expose the leaflet fusion originating from both commissures and extending through the majority of the free margins

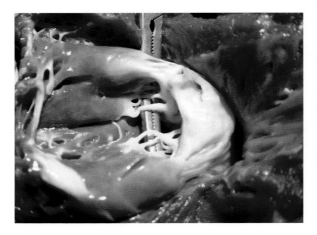

Fig. 12.3 Thickening, fusion, and retraction of the chordae tendineae in a case of rheumatic mitral stenosis

gradient increases to maintain a normal cardiac output. Series of patients followed for MS have shown a mean annual decrease in valvular area of 0.09–0.32 cm^2.[4,5] It is still a matter of discussion if the main cause of this progressive deterioration of the mitral valve is an ongoing rheumatic process or if the rheumatic event is just responsible for the initial injury and then the deformed valve further deteriorates over time by the continuous trauma inflicted by the turbulent blood flow.[6]

This gradient produces an elevation of left atrial pressures that may be as high as 25 mmHg when the mitral valvular area is 1 cm^2 (critical MS). The elevated left atrial pressure is retrogradely transmitted into the venous and capillary pulmonary bed causing dyspnea that typically exacerbates on exertion. Usually, the first symptomatic episodes appear acutely precipitated by events that increase the transmitral blood flow or produce tachycardia (which decreases the left ventricle filling time) such as physical exercise, hyperthyroidism, pregnancy (usually elicits the first symptoms in women with undiagnosed rheumatic MS), or atrial fibrillation paroxysms. These episodes can even cause acute pulmonary edema and respiratory failure in previously asymptomatic patients secondary to the acute and marked increase in left atrial pressure, especially in patients without significant pulmonary hypertension ("unprotected" MS). In a theoretical hydraulic model of MS, a twofold increase in transmitral flow produces a fourfold increase in transvalvular gradient assuming a constant mitral valve area and no changes in heart rate.[7] In real life, valve area modifies in varying degrees with cardiac output changes, and heart rates usually increase.

For a given constant cardiac output, transvalvular gradient and left atrial pressure are always higher in patients with higher heart rates.

Over time, some patients develop an increase in pulmonary arteriolar resistance that may protect their lungs from suffering pulmonary edema. This results from histological changes in the alveolar membranes, lymphatic vessels, changes in biochemical mediators production, and the response to them in the arterial and arteriolar walls. This adaptation may increase the time some patients with severe MS remain asymptomatic or may decrease their symptoms at some point during the evolution of the disease. However, this imposes a high afterload to the right ventricle that may result in tricuspid regurgitation and right atrial and ventricular dilatation and dysfunction.

Natural History

As discussed before, the landmark feature in MS conditioning the hemodynamic alterations and the clinical manifestations is the appearance and progressive increase of a pressure gradient through the mitral valve secondary to a progressive decrease in valvular orifice area. After the first episode, usually in childhood, of rheumatic carditis affecting the mitral valve, a slow but persistent deterioration of the valve starts developing. As the mitral orifice area shrinks, the hemodynamic changes produce an increase in the pulmonary wedge pressure, which in turn is responsible for most of the clinical findings usually seen in patients with severe MS.

The natural history of rheumatic MS is known from data obtained from studies carried out in the 1950s and 1960s, before cardiac surgery and modern medical treatments were available for those patients. It is not well known yet how early diagnosis and current medical management can alter the course of the disease, but is believed that it lengthens the asymptomatic interval, with symptoms appearing at older ages. It is also difficult to know if changes in the prevention and treatment of rheumatic fever have also modified the natural history of MS and the other rheumatic valvular diseases.

In patients with rheumatic MS left untreated, it has been shown that the expected evolution consists of a long and stable asymptomatic period in the first years, followed by a faster deterioration of the patient condition and leading to severe disability around a decade after the onset of symptoms[8,9] and to death at an average age of 40–50 years.[1,8]

This initial asymptomatic period after the rheumatic injury may last as much as 40 years but is usually around 15–20 years in developed countries.[10] Progression from mild to severe disability usually lasts 5–10 years more.

This pattern is shown to be significantly affected by geographical and ethnical factors. Evolution seems to be more aggressive in Polynesians, Asians, African-Americans, and the Inuits in Alaska. Socioeconomic factors have been investigated and seem to play an important role in these findings.[11–15] These variations may also be, among other reasons, due to a more severe rheumatic carditis or to repeated streptococcal infections during life.

In asymptomatic or minimally symptomatic patients, survival may be as high as 80% after 10 years with most patients remaining without progression, but when important clinical impairment develops, survival drops to less than 15% after 10 years. Important features affecting survival are atrial fibrillation and pulmonary hypertension. In patients with severe pulmonary hypertension, mean survival is around 3 years. Atrial fibrillation seems to accelerate deterioration of functional status and is a risk factor for premature death. A classic study by K.H. Olesen[16] in Denmark showed 10-year survival rate of 25% of patients with atrial fibrillation compared with 46% in patients in sinus rhythm (and 0% vs. 29% at 20 years).

Causes of death in untreated patients are congestive heart failure in 60–70%, systemic embolism in 20–30%, pulmonary embolism in 10%, and infection in 1–5%.[16,17]

In developed countries, the mean age at clinical presentation is around 40–60 years.[18,19] In less developed areas, on the contrary, the course of the disease appears to be more aggressive, with patients presenting symptoms before 20 years of age,[19] and even critical MS is seen in children during the first decade of life.

In more recent times, survival of patients with MS is longer, the main reason for that being the appearance of an effective surgical treatment that has changed natural history of the disease. However, recent data show that survival in asymptomatic patients refusing mitral valvotomy continues to be as low as 44% at 5 years.[20] This change in natural history has produced other changes; we more often see involvement of other heart valves by the rheumatic process, mainly aortic valve disease and tricuspid regurgitation.

Clinical Features

The first and most important symptom appearing in patients with rheumatic MS is exceptional dyspnea as a result of pulmonary congestion. Dyspnea can be accompanied by wheezing, cough, and in more advanced cases by orthopnea and episodes of acute pulmonary edema. Acute pulmonary edema may sometimes be the form of clinical debut in patients with MS. Symptoms may be precipitated by any condition producing tachycardia and/or an increase in transmitral blood flow as typically occurs during exercise, stress, infection, sexual intercourse, etc. Other conditions that are classically responsible for the first symptoms in the course of the disease are pregnancy and atrial fibrillation paroxysms.

As MS severity increases, patients may continue to be asymptomatic simply by reducing their physical activity. That is the reason why patients with severe MS determined by complementary tests but who remain apparently asymptomatic or with mild symptoms may need stress testing to be correctly diagnosed.

Systemic embolic events are other classical manifestations of MS (Fig. 12.4). In classical series of patients with rheumatic MS, before surgical repair and anticoagulant therapies were available, embolisms were observed in up to one fifth of patients and were responsible for about 20–30% of the mortality observed. Atrial fibrillation was present in the vast majority of these patients and its incidence is directly related with age and left atrial dilatation.

Embolic events have not been related to the anatomical or hemodynamic severity of MS and may be the first

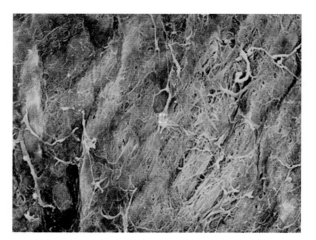

Fig. 12.4 Scanning electron microscope image of the rheumatic leaflet surface showing loss of endothelium and exposure of basal matrix. This may play a role in the high incidence of systemic embolisms even in the absence of atrial fibrillation

clinical manifestation of the disease. Any vascular territory may be affected, but around 50% of the detected systemic embolisms occur in the cerebral circulation. Patients with previous history of systemic embolism have a 25% risk of recurrence during follow-up.

Other symptoms of MS include hemoptysis, hoarseness (Ortner's syndrome, secondary to compression of the recurrent laryngeal nerve in massively dilated left atria or to dilatation of the pulmonary artery in patients with pulmonary hypertension), and signs and symptoms of right heart failure in patients with evolved pulmonary hypertension.

Physical Exam and Diagnostic Tests

Besides auscultatory findings, MS usually does not produce any clinical signs until atrial fibrillation or right heart failure occurs. Classical signs include those derived from apex palpation: a diastolic apical thrill, a tapping S1 (in pliable valves). Jugular venous pulse shows an alteration when atrial fibrillation is present or tricuspid regurgitation develops. Patients with advanced disease and low cardiac output may present with pink or purple marks in their cheeks (mitral fascies).

Auscultation in patients with MS shows many typical features. The first cardiac sound is accentuated in these patients because of the rapid rise in left ventricle pressure when the valve closes. It is directly related to the transvalvular gradient and the left atrium pressure but, as the valve loses its flexibility, gets calcified, and fuses, it may diminish and even disappear.

An opening snap of the mitral valve can be auscultated over the apex when the leaflets reach the opening position. It also requires some degree of flexibility, so it is usually accompanied by a loud S1, and it also may disappear in rigid valves. The interval between the aortic component of S2 and the opening snap is proportional to the left atrial pressure and the severity of the MS.

The typical MS diastolic murmur is low-pitched, located in the apex, and may radiate to the left axilla and lower left sternal area. The intensity of the murmur is not related with the severity of MS but its duration is. Patients in sinus rhythm present a presystolic accentuation due to the atrial contraction.

Pulmonary hypertension and right heart involvement may accentuate the pulmonary component of S2 and narrow or even erase its physiological splitting. A systolic tricuspid regurgitation murmur can also appear under these circumstances. Other auscultatory manifestations of right-sided alterations in patients with severe MS are: a systolic ejection pulmonary murmur (that diminishes with inspiration as the pulmonary artery dilates) and a pulmonary regurgitation murmur (Graham–Steell murmur that increases during inspiration).

Electrocardiography

The principal findings in severe MS are wide *p* waves ("*p* mitrale"), which are closely related with left atrial volume but not with its pressure. This is lost in patients presenting with atrial fibrillation. Right ventricular hypertrophy signs may appear in patients with pulmonary hypertension.

Chest X-Ray

The chest x-ray is usually normal in anterioposterior films because left atrial enlargement is the most frequent finding. Calcification of the mitral valve is sometimes apparent. Congestive signs can be seen in decompensated patients.

Right heart and pulmonary artery enlargement signs may be seen in patients with pulmonary hypertension.

Echocardiography

Today, transthoracic echocardiography (TTE) is the main tool for diagnosis, severity assessment, and follow-up in patients with MS. It allows a very accurate description of the diseased valve assessing and quantifying the presence of all the morphological characteristics previously described in the text: commissural fusion, thickened leaflets and chordae, retraction, calcification, and subvalvular involvement. It also adds important functional information describing leaflet mobility, valvular opening, diastolic doming, etc.

TTE can also rule out most of the entities, which have to be considered in differential diagnosis and have been mentioned before in the text. Two-dimensional examination allows detailed morphological description of the valve and subvalvular apparatus and assessment of anatomical suitability for repair (especially important when considering percutaneous balloon valvuloplasty). It also determines and quantifies the presence of mitral regurgitation (MR) and all other valvular

lesions, thus selecting those patients who should go directly for surgical repair. Left atrial volume and the presence of thrombus can also be examined. It also examines left ventricle function, pulmonary artery pressure, pericardial abnormalities, and right heart status.

Doppler study is the best tool for quantification of hemodynamic severity of obstruction in patients with MS.[21] It allows estimation of the mitral orifice area by two methods: the diastolic pressure half-time and the continuity equation method.[22–24] It is important to remark that the first may not be reliable enough in patients with other valvular lesions (mainly those with concomitant aortic regurgitation), in patients with prior valvotomy procedures, and when significant alteration in left atrium or left ventricle compliance exist.[25,26]

Transvalvular gradient may also be very accurately estimated using continuous wave Doppler signaling and the modified Bernoulli equation across the valve. However, this measure may be seriously affected by heart rate, which is especially important in patients in atrial fibrillation.

TTE is also employed in exercise testing in these patients.[27,28] Doppler registration of both transmitral and transtricuspid flow velocities determine how transvalvular gradient and pulmonary artery pressure modify with exercise.

Transesophageal echocardiography (TEE) produces better quality images and more accurate measures although it is currently not recommended for all patients since this usually does not traduce an increase in accuracy. TEE is indicated when transthoracic examination is not enough for correct diagnosis, severity assessment, or management decision making guidance. Another indication for considering transesophageal examination is a history of previous embolic events, in order to determine the presence of left atrial thrombus, especially if balloon valvuloplasty is being considered.

Intervention

Closed Surgical Commissurotomy

The original idea of mitral valvotomy first came out in 1902 from Sir Lauder Brunton[29] and the first procedure performed in a patient was carried out in 1923 by Levine and Cutler using a specifically designed transapical knife.[30] Other closed procedures, using different instruments and frequently with the help of the surgeon's finger through the left atrial appendage, were developed to open stenotic valves in subsequent years.[31-33]

With the development and increasing availability of cardiopulmonary bypass systems, open procedures began in the 1950s but really did not replace closed operations until the late 1960s. The first successful mitral valve replacement was reported in 1961 by Starr and Edwards in Oregon using their mechanical prosthesis.[34]

Currently, the most commonly employed technique is the transapical commissurotomy using a Tubbs dilator introduced through a purse-string suture at the left ventricle apex. The instrument's tip through the mitral valve is controlled using the right index finger, which is introduced through the tip of the left atrial appendage through another purse-string suture. Care must be taken that the dilator blades are opened against the leaflets and not against the commissures. Several successive dilatations are performed increasing the opening distance of the tip of the instrument, allowing the heart to recover before repeating the next maneuver. Initial opening should be attempted with the surgeon's finger because sometimes this can be enough to remove valvular obstruction, with no further interventions needed. If a dilator is finally required, the initial opening diameter should be set around 2.5 cm, and then increasing slowly afterwards until reaching a 4-cm aperture. Attention must be focused to detect significant mitral regurgitation between successive dilatations and if it is identified the procedure should be interrupted. This procedure as described can be performed without the need for cardiopulmonary bypass.

Closed techniques have been almost completely abandoned in developed countries, where they have been replaced by the open surgical commissurotomy and the percutaneous balloon valvuloplasty (PMBV). Both procedures have consistently showed their superiority over closed commissurotomy in large series[35,36] and clinical trials.[37]

Due to its lower cost, the closed surgical commissurotomy is still a very valuable tool in developing regions, where younger patients with more pliable valves are frequently treated with good results.

Open Surgical Commissurotomy

Open surgical commissurotomy is the preferred technique for surgical correction of MS in developed

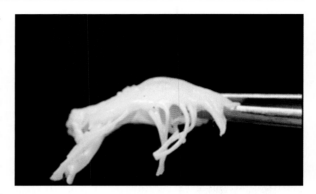

Fig. 12.5 This picture shows the rigidity of the leaflets in rheumatic MS. The entire leaflet with the chordae is held with the tip of the forceps and keeps its shape due to increased rigidity

countries. It is performed under cardiopulmonary bypass and usually with cardiac arrest. It allows the surgeon to open the valve under direct vision and the immediate assessment of the anatomical result. Functional testing can also be carried out on the repaired valve before ending the procedure.

This technique is applicable in patients not suitable for the percutaneous valvotomy, like those with severely fibrotic or calcified valves (Fig. 12.5). It also allows the surgeon to add any other procedure that may be needed, e.g. extraction of all left atrial thrombus and left atrial appendage amputation, correction of concomitant MR by means of mitral annuloplasty or other techniques, and correction of other simultaneous lesions that may be present aortic regurgitation (AR), tricuspid regurgitation (TR), or coronary disease.

This operation is usually performed through a median sternotomy, but it might also be accomplished through a right anterolateral thoracotomy.

Assessing the characteristics of the subvalvular apparatus is often only possible after some degree of leaflet and commissure fusion is lysed (Fig. 12.6). Heavily calcified leaflet and commissures can be decalcified with caution with the aid of a rongeur. Sometimes, papillary muscles must be incised and partially divided when chordae are shortened. Commissural incisions must usually leave a 2–3 mm edge to the annulus. Other techniques that may be needed include creation of neochordae and lengthening of the anterior leaflet.[38]

This procedure almost always results in a mitral valve area greater than 2 cm^2 and even >3 cm^2 in 37% of patients with good morphological characteristics in experienced centers.[39]

These techniques have shown excellent results in long-term follow-up series, with a low restenosis rate

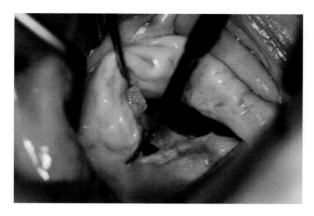

Fig. 12.6 After opening the fused commissures, inspection of the subvalvular apparatus is possible. In this picture, fused and retracted chordae and papillary muscles are divided with the scalpel

and up to 81% of patients having a mitral valve area (MVA) >2 cm² after 8.5 years[39] and 96–98% freedom from reintervention at 7–10 years.[39,40] Comparative trials, however, have not shown significant advantage when compared with PMBV.[37,41,42] The fact that PMBV offers a less aggressive alternative – avoiding thoracotomy or sternotomy – and obtains similar long-term results, makes it, at this time, the preferred option for patients that are suitable for both procedures.

Percutaneous Mitral Balloon Valvuloplasty

Percutaneous transvenous mitral balloon valvuloplasty (PMBV) is currently recommended as the first-line treatment in MS for all patients when available and no contraindications for the procedure exist. It was introduced and developed by Inoue in Japan in 1984.[43] The mechanism by which PMBV works is the same employed in closed surgical commissurotomy procedures. It generates a minimally invasive mechanical dilatation of the valve resulting in splitting of the fused commissures.

The most usually employed approach is the transseptal technique. It consists of advancing the catheter "over the wire" across the interatrial septum after transseptal puncture from a percutaneous femoral vein catheterization. After dilatation of the orifice in the septum, either a large Inoue balloon catheter (single balloon technique or Inoue technique) or two smaller balloon catheters (double-balloon technique, inflated simultaneously, 15–20 mm each) are advanced through the mitral orifice and the valve is dilated during their inflation. The most

frequently used technique worldwide nowadays is the single-balloon approach although both have showed similar results. The balloon has an hour-glass shape and has 23–28 mm size. The single balloon technique has several advantages for some authors as: reduced profile of the device, easier maneuverability, and less risk of ventricular perforation (stiff wire not necessary). Another advantage of the single-balloon technique is the possibility of progressive sequential dilatation of the mitral orifice using increasing balloon sizes.[44] This technique usually produces, on average, an increase in valvular area from 1 to 2 cm² and a drop of transvalvular gradient from 18 to 6 mmHg.

A metallic and reusable valvulotome has been designed and seems to provide comparable results.[45] This instrument may reduce the costs of the procedure and spread its application to less developed areas.[46,47]

The mitral valve morphology is assessed before the procedure by transthoracic echocardiography and is considered favorable for the technique if the semi-quantitative Wilkins score is less than 8[48] (Table 12.1). This score takes into account leaflet rigidity, thickening, valvular calcification, and subvalvular disease. Each one of these items is evaluated and a value between 1 and 4 is assigned. Higher scores predict worse short- and long-term results and increase the risk for developing acute MR. Other similar scoring systems exist and have shown a good performance in clinical studies, predicting outcome and development of MR after the procedure.[49] Patients with atrial fibrillation should undergo transesophageal examination before attempting the PMBV, which is contraindicated in the presence of left atrial thrombus.

Published results after PMBV show an immediate increase in estimated mitral valve area (MVA) from an initial around 0.8–1.2 cm² to 1.8–2.2 cm².[50,51] These results are strongly influenced by the preprocedure echo score. Immediate success is usually defined as MVA ≥ 1.5 cm² and less than grade 2/4 mitral regurgitation.

The most frequent complications after the procedure are mitral regurgitation and persistent atrial septal defect, with an incidence of around 15% and 20%, respectively.[50–54] The incidence of mitral regurgitation after PMBV is relatively high in absolute terms but severe mitral regurgitation requiring surgery occurs in 1–2% of cases. Atrial septal defects are frequently detected by color Doppler echocardiography immediately after the procedure, but usually are not hemodynamically significant and the majority of them tend to decrease during follow-up or even disappear.

Table 12.1 Determinants of the echocardiographic mitral valve score (From Wilkins et al.[48] Used with permission.)

Grade	Mobility	Subvalvular thickening	Thickening	Calcification
1	Highly mobile valve with only leaflet tips restricted	Minimal thickening just below the mitral leaflets	Leaflets near normal in thickness (4–5 mm)	A single area of increased echo brightness
2	Leaflet mid and base portions have normal mobility	Thickening of the chordal structures extending up to one third of the chordal length	Midleaflets normal, considerable thickening of margins (5–8 mm)	Scattered areas of brightness confined to leaflet margins
3	Valve continues to move forward in diastole, mainly from the base	Thickening extending to the distal third of the chords	Thickening extending through the entire leaflet (5–8 mm)	Brightness extending into the midportion of the leaflets
4	No or minimal forward movement of the leaflets in diastole	Extensive thickening and shortening of all chordal structures extending down to the papillary muscles	Considerable thickening of all leaflet tissue (>8–10 mm)	Extensive brightness throughout much of the leaflet tissue

Severe complications after the procedure are relatively infrequent, especially in patients with good morphological scores. Mortality is less than 1% and stroke incidence is around 1%, as is the incidence of cardiac tamponade.[50–54] These results are markedly operator-dependent.

In the long term, as in surgical commissurotomy, the main issue affecting the results is restenosis. The restenosis rate is reported to be between 33% and 39% at 7 years after the procedure.[55,56] In patients with good morphological characteristics for PMBV, as defined by a Wilkins score ≤8, restenosis rates have been reported to be as low as 11% at 6.5 years of mean follow-up.[51] Table 12.2 lists contraindications to percutaneous mitral balloon valvuloplasty.[57]

Event-free survival (cardiac death, NYHA class III or IV, and redo-PMBV or MVR) after PMBV is 61% at 10 years in patients with initial success of the technique.[58] Other series communicate a 32% in patients with Wilkins scores ≤8 and 22% in patients with scores >8 at 12 years.[59]

Predictive factors for restenosis and worse outcome are advanced age, poor immediate postprocedure MVA(<2 cm²), more than 2/4 mitral regurgitation after PMBV, Wilkins echocardiographic score >8, atrial fibrillation, and advanced NYHA and/or pulmonary artery pressure after the completion of the procedure.[51,55,56,60–63]

Another interesting use of PMBV is in the setting of patients with prior open or closed surgical commissurotomy, who, after years from surgery develop significant restenosis and may particularly benefit from avoiding the risk that carries a reintervention. The success rate of the procedure under these circumstances

Table 12.2 Contraindications to percutaneous mitral balloon valvuloplasty (Modified from the 2007-ESC guidelines.[57] Used with permission.)

Mitral valve area >1.5 cm²
Left atrial thrombus
More than mild MR
Severe or bicommisural calcification
Absence of commissural fusion
Severe concomitant aortic valve disease or severe combined TS and TR
Concomitant condition requiring cardiac surgery

MR mitral regurgitation, *TR* tricuspid regurgitation, *TS* tricuspid stenosis

has been shown not to differ significantly from the "de novo" intervention and is around 82–93%.[64–66] Longer follow-up series show worse results than primary PMBV, with event-free survival rates (as defined previously) at 10 years of 54%.[64,67,68]

A similar situation represents the repeated PMBV in patients developing restenosis after the initial procedure, with an initial success rate (MVA ≥ 1.5 cm² and MR <2/4) of 91% and around 69% of patients in NYHA class I or II and free from reintervention at 5 years.[69]

Another situation of particular interest is the treatment of pregnant women, who, as was discussed earlier, are especially at risk for clinical worsening and serious complications due to their particular physiologic hemodynamic situation.[70] These patients and their fetuses are in greater risk for death and adverse events, especially during labor and delivery.[71] Many patients are first diagnosed of rheumatic MS during pregnancy, and some of them may require treatment on an emergency basis.

Both surgical (open and closed) and percutaneous treatments have been used in this setting with similarly good results, but surgical interventions have been associated with higher maternal and fetal mortality, making PMBV the first option to treat these women whenever possible.[72-75] PMBV should preferably be avoided during the first trimester, and should be performed minimizing fluoroscopy time and using protective abdominopelvic radiation shielding.

Indication

Severity of MS is asserted by several variables, as there is not a single piece of information that can correctly judge its severity and classify all patients. MS severity

assessment is then based on the reunion of hemodynamic and clinical findings and natural history data. Guidelines from the *European Society of Cardiology* (ESC)[57] and from the *American Heart Association/American College of Cardiology* (AHA/ACC)[76] are frequently revised and published to help physicians and surgeons with the management of patients with rheumatic MS. The most recent management algorithms proposed by these two societies are shown in Figs. 12.7 and 12.8, which show the current recommendations from the ESC and the ACC/AHA to catalog MS severity according to valve area, transvalvular gradient, and pulmonary hypertension measurements.

When considering intervention, the first step is to differentiate patients based on the presence of symptoms. Asymptomatic patients with severe MS (valvular area less than 1.5 cm²) should not undergo surgical repair or replacement in a general basis. Percutaneous

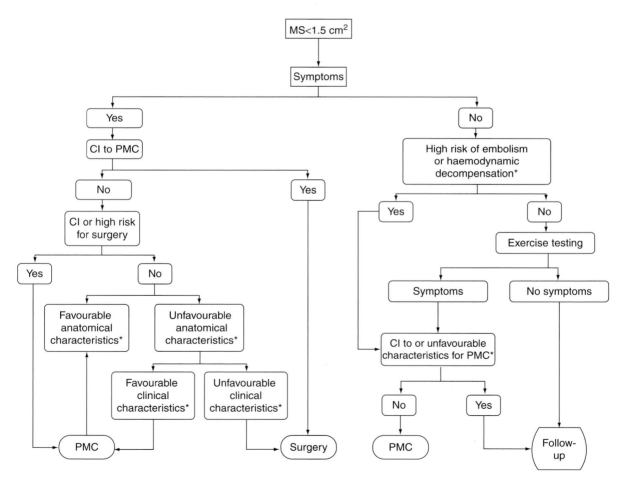

Fig. 12.7 ESC recommendations for management of patients with mitral stenosis. *MS* mitral stenosis, *CI* contraindication, *PMC* percutaneous mitral commissurotomy. *See Table 12.3 for description of these characteristics (From Vahanian et al.[57] Used with permission.)

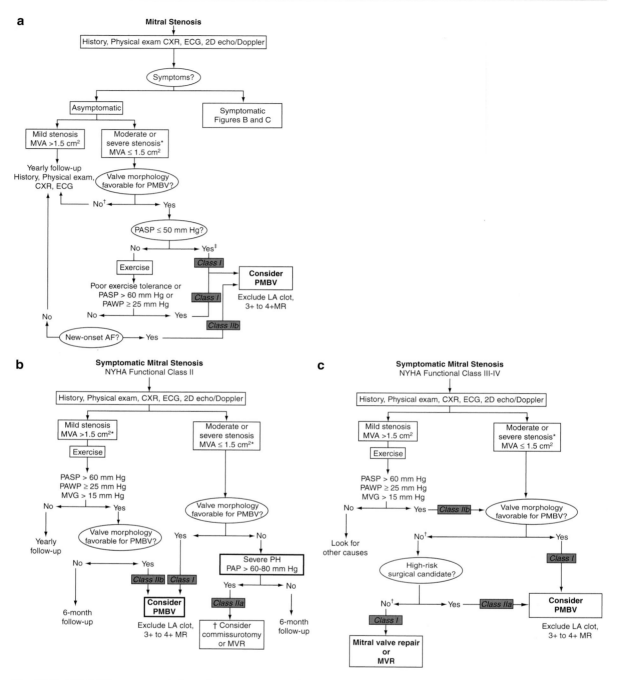

Fig. 12.8 *AHA/ACC* recommendations for management of patients with asymptomatic mitral stenosis (**a**), patients with NYHA class II symptoms (**b**) and those with class III or IV symptoms (**c**). *MVA* mitral valve area, *PAWP* pulmonary artery wedge pressure, *PASP* pulmonary artery systolic pressure, *CXR* chest X-ray, *ECG* electrocardiography, *LA* left atrial, *MR* mitral regurgitation, *MVG* mean mitral valve pressure gradient, *MVR* mitral valve replacement, *NYHA* New York Heart Association, 2D two-dimensional. †It is controversial as to which patients with less favorable valve morphology should undergo percutaneous mitral balloon valvotomy (PMBV) rather than mitral valve surgery (From Bonow et al.[57] Used with permission.)

Table 12.3 Indications for percutaneous mitral balloon valvuloplasty in mitral stenosis with valvular area <1.5 cm² (From the 2007-ESC guidelines.[57] Used with permission.)

	Class
Symptomatic patients with favorable characteristics for PMBV[a]	IB
Symptomatic patients with contraindication or high risk for surgery	IC
As initial treatment in symptomatic patients with unfavorable anatomy but otherwise favorable clinical characteristics[a]	IIaC
Asymptomatic patients with favorable characteristics and high thrombo-embolic risk or high risk of hemodynamic decompensation:	
Previous history of embolism	IIaC
Dense spontaneous contrast in the left atrium	IIaC
Recent or paroxysmal atrial fibrillation	IIaC
Systolic pulmonary pressure >50 mmHg at rest	IIaC
Need for major noncardiac surgery	IIaC
Desire of pregnancy	IIaC

[a]Favorable characteristics for PMBV can be defined by the absence of several of the following: (1) clinical characteristics: old age, history of commissurotomy, NYHA IV, atrial fibrillation, and severe pulmonary hypertension; (2) Anatomical characteristics: echo score >8, Cormier score 3, very small mitral valve area, severe tricuspid regurgitation.

mitral balloon valvuloplasty (PMBV) should be considered under these circumstances in patients on high risk for embolic events or hemodynamic decompensation when favorable anatomy and no contraindications for the technique are present (Table 12.3). Asymptomatic patients without these risk factors and a positive exercise test may also undergo PMBV if there is no contraindication and a favorable anatomy exists. The 2006-ACC/AHA recommendations also consider new onset of atrial fibrillation as a class IIb recommendation for PMBV in anatomical favorable cases even with negative exercise testing.

When symptoms occur in patients with severe MS, the indication for correction is established and PMBV should be the preferred method if available. All patients with contraindication for PMBV should be considered for surgical correction. Symptomatic patients who are good candidates for both techniques should be preferably sent for PMBV unless unfavorable anatomical and clinical characteristics for the procedure are present.

At last, although not frequent, there are symptomatic patients with mild MS according to echocardiography. The 2006-ACC/AHA guidelines recommend performing an exercise test in these patients. If pulmonary artery systolic pressure goes higher than 60 mmHg, pulmonary artery wedge pressure greater than or equal to 25 mmHg, or transvalvular gradient greater than 15 mmHg, PMBV should be considered as a class IIb recommendation if valve morphology is favorable. Those patients with unfavorable anatomy for PMBV and a positive exercise test are followed every 6 months. Patients with a negative exercise test should be yearly followed.

References

1. Rowe JC, Bland EF, Sprague HB, et al. The course of mitral stenosis without surgery: ten- and twenty-year perspectives. *Ann Intern Med.* 1960;52:741-749.
2. Wood P. An appreciation of mitral stenosis. I. Clinical features. *Br Med J.* 1954;1(4870):1051-1063.
3. Heller SJ, Carleton RA. Abnormal left ventricular contraction in patients with mitral stenosis. *Circulation.* 1970;42(6):1099-1110.
4. Dubin AA, March HW, Cohn K, et al. Longitudinal hemodynamic and clinical study of mitral stenosis. *Circulation.* 1971;44(3):381-389.
5. Gordon SP, Douglas PS, Come PC, et al. Two-dimensional and Doppler echocardiographic determinants of the natural history of mitral valve narrowing in patients with rheumatic mitral stenosis: implications for follow-up. *J Am Coll Cardiol.* 1992;19(5):968-973.
6. Selzer A, Cohn KE. Natural history of mitral stenosis: a review. *Circulation.* 1972;45(4):878-890.
7. Gorlin R, Gorlin SG. Hydraulic formula for calculation of the area of the stenotic mitral valve, other cardiac valves, and central circulatory shunts. I. *Am Heart J.* 1951;41(1):1-29.
8. Rapaport E. Natural history of aortic and mitral valve disease. *Am J Cardiol.* 1975;35(2):221-227.
9. Wood P. An appreciation of mitral stenosis. I. Clinical features. *Br Med J.* 1954;1(4870):1051-1063.
10. Bland EF, Duckett JT. Rheumatic fever and rheumatic heart disease; a twenty year report on 1000 patients followed since childhood. *Circulation.* 1951;4(6):836-843.
11. Angelino PF, Levi V, Brusca a, et al. Mitral commissurotomy in the younger age group. *Am Heart J.* 1956;51(6):916-925.
12. al-Bahrani IR, Thamer MA, al-Omeri MM, et al. Rheumatic heart disease in the young in Iraq. *Br Heart J.* 1966;28(6):824-828.

13. Cherian G, Vytilingam KI, Sukumar IP, et al. Mitral valvotomy in young patients. *Br Heart J.* 1964;26:157-166.
14. Manteuffel-Szoege L, Nowicki J, Wasniewska M, et al. Mitral commissurotomy. Results in 1700 cases. *J Cardiovasc Surg (Torino).* 1970;11(5):350-354.
15. Roy SB, Gopinath N. Mitral stenosis. *Circulation.* 1968; 38(1 Suppl):68-76.
16. Olesen KH. The natural history of 271 patients with mitral stenosis under medical treatment. *Br Heart J.* 1962;24: 349-357.
17. Roberts WC, Perloff JK. Mitral valvular disease. A clinicopathologic survey of the conditions causing the mitral valve to function abnormally. *Ann Intern Med.* 1972;77(6):939-975.
18. Carroll JD, Feldman T. Percutaneous mitral balloon valvotomy and the new demographics of mitral stenosis. *JAMA.* 1993;270(14):1731-1736.
19. Selzer A, Cohn KE. Natural history of mitral stenosis: a review. *Circulation.* 1972;45(4):878-890.
20. Horstkotte D, Niehues R, Strauer BE. Pathomorphological aspects, aetiology and natural history of acquired mitral valve stenosis. *Eur Heart J.* 1991;12(Suppl B):55-60.
21. Faletra F, Pezzano A Jr, Fusco R, et al. Measurement of mitral valve area in mitral stenosis: four echocardiographic methods compared with direct measurement of anatomic orifices. *J Am Coll Cardiol.* 1996;28(5):1190-1197.
22. Hatle L, Brubakk A, Tromsdal A, et al. Noninvasive assessment of pressure drop in mitral stenosis by Doppler ultrasound. *Br Heart J.* 1978;40(2):131-140.
23. Hatle L, Angelsen B, Tromsdal A. Noninvasive assessment of atrioventricular pressure half-time by Doppler ultrasound. *Circulation.* 1979;60(5):1096-1104.
24. Nakatani S, Masuyama T, Kodama K, et al. Value and limitations of Doppler echocardiography in the quantification of stenotic mitral valve area: comparison of the pressure half-time and the continuity equation methods. *Circulation.* 1988; 77(1):78-85.
25. Thomas JD, Wilkins GT, Choong CY, et al. Inaccuracy of mitral pressure half-time immediately after percutaneous mitral valvotomy. Dependence on transmitral gradient and left atrial and ventricular compliance. *Circulation.* 1988; 78(4):980-993.
26. Flachskampf FA, Weyman AE, Guerrero JL, et al. Influence of orifice geometry and flow rate on effective valve area: an in vitro study. *J Am Coll Cardiol.* 1990;15(5): 1173-1180.
27. Leavitt JI, Coats MH, Falk RH. Effects of exercise on transmitral gradient and pulmonary artery pressure in patients with mitral stenosis or a prosthetic mitral valve: a Doppler echocardiographic study. *J Am Coll Cardiol.* 1991;17(7): 1520-1526.
28. Lev EI, Sagie A, Vaturi M, et al. Value of exercise echocardiography in rheumatic mitral stenosis with and without significant mitral regurgitation. *Am J Cardiol.* 2004; 93(8): 1060-1063.
29. Brunton L, Edin M. Preliminary note on the possibility of treating mitral stenosis by surgical methods. *Lancet.* 1902;1:352.
30. Cutler E, Levine S. Cardiotomy and valvulotomy for mitral stenosis: experimental observations and clinical notes concerning an operated case with recovery. *Boston Med Surg J.* 1923;188:1023.
31. Austen WG, Wooler GH. Surgical treatment of mitral stenosis by the transventricular approach with a mechanical dilator. *N Engl J Med.* 1960;263:661-665.
32. Harken DE, Black H. Improved valvuloplasty for mitral stenosis, with a discussion of multivalvular disease. *N Engl J Med.* 1955;253(16):669-678.
33. Souttar H. The surgical treatment of mitral stenosis. *Br Med J.* 1925;2:603.
34. Starr A, Edwards ML. Mitral replacement: clinical experience with a ball-valve prosthesis. *Ann Surg.* 1961;154: 726-740.
35. Hickey MS, Blackstone EH, Kirklin JW, et al. Outcome probabilities and life history after surgical mitral commissurotomy: implications for balloon commissurotomy. *J Am Coll Cardiol.* 1991;17(1):29-42.
36. Commerford PJ, Hastie T, Beck W. Closed mitral valvotomy: actuarial analysis of results in 654 patients over 12 years and analysis of preoperative predictors of long-term survival. *Ann Thorac Surg.* 1982;33(5):473-479.
37. Ben FM, Ayari M, Maatouk F, et al. Percutaneous balloon versus surgical closed and open mitral commissurotomy: seven-year follow-up results of a randomized trial. *Circulation.* 1998;97(3):245-250.
38. Duran CM, Gometza B, Saad E. Valve repair in rheumatic mitral disease: an unsolved problem. *J Card Surg.* 1994;9(2 Suppl):282-285.
39. Antunes MJ, Vieira H, de Ferrao OJ. Open mitral commissurotomy: the "golden standard". *J Heart Valve Dis.* 2000; 9(4):472-477.
40. Choudhary SK, Dhareshwar J, Govil a, et al. Open mitral commissurotomy in the current era: indications, technique, and results. *Ann Thorac Surg.* 2003;75(1):41-46.
41. Cotrufo M, Renzulli a, Ismeno G, et al. Percutaneous mitral commissurotomy versus open mitral commissurotomy: a comparative study. *Eur J Cardiothorac Surg.* 1999;15(5): 646-651.
42. Reyes VP, Raju BS, Wynne J, et al. Percutaneous balloon valvuloplasty compared with open surgical commissurotomy for mitral stenosis. *N Engl J Med.* 1994;331(15): 961-967.
43. Inoue K, Owaki T, Nakamura T, et al. Clinical application of transvenous mitral commissurotomy by a new balloon catheter. *J Thorac Cardiovasc Surg.* 1984;87(3):394-402.
44. Fawzy ME, Mimish L, Sivanandam V, et al. Advantage of Inoue balloon catheter in mitral balloon valvotomy: experience with 220 consecutive patients. *Cathet Cardiovasc Diagn.* 1996;38(1):9-14.
45. Cribier A, Eltchaninoff H, Koning R, et al. Percutaneous mechanical mitral commissurotomy with a newly designed metallic valvulotome: immediate results of the initial experience in 153 patients. *Circulation.* 1999;99(6):793-799.
46. Arora R, Kalra GS, Singh S, et al. Non-surgical mitral commissurotomy using metallic commissurotome. *Indian Heart J.* 1998;50(1):91-95.
47. Harikrishnan S, Bhat a, Tharakan J, et al. Percutaneous transvenous mitral commissurotomy using metallic commissurotome: long-term follow-up results. *J Invasive Cardiol.* 2006; 18(2):54-58.
48. Wilkins GT, Weyman AE, Abascal VM, et al. Percutaneous balloon dilatation of the mitral valve: an analysis of echocardiographic variables related to outcome and the mechanism of dilatation. *Br Heart J.* 1988;60(4):299-308.

49. Padial LR, Freitas N, Sagie a, et al. Echocardiography can predict which patients will develop severe mitral regurgitation after percutaneous mitral valvulotomy. *J Am Coll Cardiol.* 1996;27(5):1225-1231.

50. Reid CL, Otto CM, Davis KB, et al. Influence of mitral valve morphology on mitral balloon commissurotomy: immediate and six-month results from the NHLBI Balloon Valvuloplasty Registry. *Am Heart J.* 1992;124(3):657-665.

51. Fawzy ME, Fadel B, Al-Sergani H, et al. Long-term results (up to 16.5 years) of mitral balloon valvuloplasty in a series of 518 patients and predictors of long-term outcome. *J Interv Cardiol.* 2007;20(1):66-72.

52. Ishikura F, Nagata S, Yasuda S, et al. Residual atrial septal perforation after percutaneous transvenous mitral commissurotomy with Inoue balloon catheter. *Am Heart J.* 1990;120(4): 873-878.

53. Yamabe T, Nagata S, Ishikura F, et al. Influence of intra-balloon pressure on development of severe mitral regurgitation after percutaneous transvenous mitral commissurotomy. *Cathet Cardiovasc Diagn.* 1994;31(4):270-276.

54. Casale P, Block PC, óShea JP, et al. Atrial septal defect after percutaneous mitral balloon valvuloplasty: immediate results and follow-up. *J Am Coll Cardiol.* 1990;15(6):1300-1304.

55. Kang DH, Park SW, Song JK, et al. Long-term clinical and echocardiographic outcome of percutaneous mitral valvuloplasty: randomized comparison of Inoue and double-balloon techniques. *J Am Coll Cardiol.* 2000;35(1):169-175.

56. Hernandez R, Banuelos C, Alfonso F, et al. Long-term clinical and echocardiographic follow-up after percutaneous mitral valvuloplasty with the Inoue balloon. *Circulation.* 1999;99(12):1580-1586.

57. Vahanian A, Baumgartner H, Bax J, et al. Guidelines on the management of valvular heart disease: the Task Force on the Management of Valvular Heart Disease of the European Society of Cardiology. *Eur Heart J.* 2007;28(2): 230-268.

58. Iung B, Garbarz E, Michaud P, et al. Late results of percutaneous mitral commissurotomy in a series of 1024 patients. Analysis of late clinical deterioration: frequency, anatomic findings, and predictive factors. *Circulation.* 1999;99(25): 3272-3278.

59. Palacios IF, Sanchez PL, Harrell LC, et al. Which patients benefit from percutaneous mitral balloon valvuloplasty? Prevalvuloplasty and postvalvuloplasty variables that predict long-term outcome. *Circulation.* 2002;105(12): 1465-1471.

60. Vahanian A, Iung B. Percutaneous mitral balloon commissurotomy: a useful and necessary treatment for the western population. *Eur Heart J.* 2000;21(20):1651-1652.

61. Iung B, Vahanian A. The long-term outcome of balloon valvuloplasty for mitral stenosis. *Curr Cardiol Rep.* 2002; 4(2):118-124.

62. Chmielak Z, Kruk M, Demkow M, et al. Long-term follow-up of patients with percutaneous mitral commissurotomy. *Kardiol Pol.* 2008;66(5):525-530. discussion.

63. Ben-Farhat M, Betbout F, Gamra H, et al. Predictors of long-term event-free survival and of freedom from restenosis after percutaneous balloon mitral commissurotomy. *Am Heart J.* 2001;142(6):1072-1079.

64. Fawzy ME, Hassan W, Shoukri M, et al. Immediate and long-term results of mitral balloon valvotomy for restenosis following previous surgical or balloon mitral commissurotomy. *Am J Cardiol.* 2005;96(7):971-975.

65. Neumayer U, Schmidt HK, Fassbender D, et al. Balloon mitral valvotomy after surgical commissurotomy: clinical and hemodynamic results of a large, single-center study. *J Heart Valve Dis.* 2004;13(5):760-765.

66. Serra A, Bonan R, Lefevre T, et al. Balloon mitral commissurotomy for mitral restenosis after surgical commissurotomy. *Am J Cardiol.* 1993;71(15):1311-1315.

67. Chmielak Z, Ruzyllo W, Demkow M, et al. Late results of percutaneous balloon mitral commissurotomy in patients with restenosis after surgical commissurotomy compared to patients with 'de-novo' stenosis. *J Heart Valve Dis.* 2002; 11(4):509-516.

68. Iung B, Garbarz E, Michaud P, et al. Percutaneous mitral commissurotomy for restenosis after surgical commissurotomy: late efficacy and implications for patient selection. *J Am Coll Cardiol.* 2000;35(5):1295-1302.

69. Iung B, Garbarz E, Michaud P, et al. Immediate and mid-term results of repeat percutaneous mitral commissurotomy for restenosis following earlier percutaneous mitral commissurotomy. *Eur Heart J.* 2000;21(20):1683-1689.

70. Elkayam U, Bitar F. Valvular heart disease and pregnancy part I: native valves. *J Am Coll Cardiol.* 2005; 46(2):223-230.

71. Silversides CK, Colman JM, Sermer M, et al. Cardiac risk in pregnant women with rheumatic mitral stenosis. *Am J Cardiol.* 2003;91(11):1382-1385.

72. Fawzy ME, Kinsara AJ, Stefadouros M, et al. Long-Term outcome of mitral balloon valvotomy in pregnant women. *J Heart Valve Dis.* 2001;10(2):153-157.

73. Esteves CA, Munoz JS, Braga S, et al. Immediate and long-term follow-up of percutaneous balloon mitral valvuloplasty in pregnant patients with rheumatic mitral stenosis. *Am J Cardiol.* 2006;98(6):812-816.

74. de Andrade J, Maldonado M, Pontes JS, et al. The role of mitral valve balloon valvuloplasty in the treatment of rheumatic mitral valve stenosis during pregnancy. *Rev Esp Cardiol.* 2001;54(5):573-579.

75. de Souza JA, Martinez EE Jr, Ambrose JA, et al. Percutaneous balloon mitral valvuloplasty in comparison with open mitral valve commissurotomy for mitral stenosis during pregnancy. *J Am Coll Cardiol.* 2001;37(3):900-903.

76. Bonow RO, Carabello BA, Chatterjee K, et al. ACC/AHA 2006 guidelines for the management of patients with valvular heart disease: a report of the American College of Cardiology/ American Heart Association Task Force on Practice Guidelines (writing Committee to Revise the 1998 guidelines for the management of patients with valvular heart disease) developed in collaboration with the Society of Cardiovascular Anesthesiologists endorsed by the Society for Cardiovascular Angiography and Interventions and the Society of Thoracic Surgeons. *J Am Coll Cardiol.* 2006; 48(3):1-148.

Part III

Other Conditions

Atrial Fibrillation: Non Surgical Management

13

Chee W. Khoo and Gregory Y.H. Lip

Introduction

Atrial fibrillation (AF) is the most common sustained cardiac arrhythmia in clinical practice. The prevalence of AF increases with age. Indeed, there is one in four chance for both men and women aged 40 and above to develop AF during their life.[1] With the increase in aging population, AF has become a major condition that requires extra resources in its management as well as the complications associated with it.

AF is often associated with increase in mortality and morbidity from thromboembolic events including stroke, heart failure, and impaired quality of life. Many of the patients do not get hospitalized until they develop complications. Hence, much of the management of AF is mainly community-based.

AF is associated with several cardiac causes, which include coronary artery disease, hypertension, valvular heart disease, cardiomyopathy, and pericarditis. The noncardiac causes of AF include hyperthyroidism, electrolytes imbalance, hypoxia, diabetes, alcohol, and drugs (caffeine, cocaine). There is also a strong family history associated with AF, with a risk of as high as 30%.[2]

Pathophysiology and Electrophysiology

There are extensive literature reviews on the pathophysiology and electrophysiology of AF, and a detailed treatise is beyond the scope of this chapter.

For many years, AF was thought to be due to multiple re-entrant wavelets on animal studies, but more recent studies have emphasized the concept of a focus point with stable re-entrant circuit of short cycle length or unstable re-entrant of short cycle length that "drives" the atrium too rapidly and thus causes the atria to fibrillate. The focus points are often near one or more of the pulmonary veins.[3,4]

Patients in AF lack the normal atrial systolic function and the contribution to diastolic ventricular filling, and the ventricles usually respond with an irregular rhythm and fast rate. This results in impaired cardiac function and while some patients with AF are asymptomatic, some patients report symptoms of reduced exercise tolerance, palpitations, chest pain, breathlessness and dizziness, as well as syncope. The effect of reduced stroke volume and cardiac output is more profound in patients with structural heart disease.

AF also causes changes on the myocardium and progressive dilatation of left atrium. Poorly controlled AF rates result in ventricular dilatation and impaired systolic function, the so-called "tachycardia-induced cardiomyopathy."

The lack of atrial systolic function also promotes thrombogenesis secondary to intra-atrial stasis of blood, particularly within the left atrial appendage. The risk of thromboembolism is increased with structural heart disease and cardiovascular risk factors.

G.Y.H. Lip (✉)
University of Birmingham Centre for Cardiovascular Sciences, City Hospital, Birmingham, West Midlands, UK
e-mail: g.y.h.lip@bham.ac.uk

R.S. Bonser et al. (eds.), *Mitral Valve Surgery*,
DOI: 10.1007/978-1-84996-426-5_13, © Springer-Verlag London Limited 2011

Furthermore, abnormalities of blood constituents – coagulation parameters, platelets, inflammation, etc. – are present, fulfilling Virchow's triad for thrombogenesis, resulting in AF conferring a prothrombotic or hypercoagulable state.[5]

Clinical Classification

AF can be easily recognized in most of the patients by using electrocardiogram (ECG). The lack of P waves, and the presence of rapid, irregular fibrillatory waves and irregular ventricular response on the ECG are used to diagnose AF. Assessment of patients includes a thorough history taking and physical examination, with emphasis on complications and comorbidities of AF.

The clinical presentation of AF is now generally classified according to the temporal pattern of presentation,[6] as follows: (i) recent onset (within 48 h); (ii) paroxysmal; (iii) persistent (duration 7 days or more); (iv) permanent (duration greater than 1 year or refractory to cardioversion attempts). This simple classification (Fig. 13.1) merely offers approach to the likely time-course of AF and may help guide the approach to management and treatment objectives. In reality, however, the management of patients with AF should be guided by many considerations, including symptoms, hemodynamic stability, and the associated co-morbidities (e.g., hypertension and heart failure).

Pharmacological Agents

There are numerous pharmacological agents that can be used to restore and maintain sinus rhythm as well as to control ventricular rate in AF. There are different modes of actions depending on which group of drugs that a clinician chooses to use.

The most commonly used classification to describe various drugs is the Vaughan-Williams classification (Table 13.1).

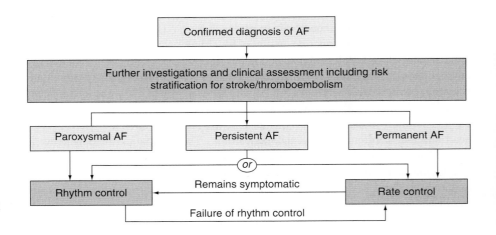

Fig. 13.1 Patterns of atrial fibrillation

Table 13.1 Vaughan-Williams classification of antiarrhythmic drugs

	Action	Examples
Class Ia	Prolongs the action potential	Disopyramide, Procainamide, Quinidine
Class Ib	Shortens the action potential	Lidocaine, Mexiletine
Class Ic	No significant effect on action potential	Flecainide, Propafenone
Class II	Beta adregenic blockers	Propranolol, Atenolol
Class III	Potassium channel blockers that prolong repolarization	Amiodarone, Bretylium, Dofetilide, Ibutilide, Sotalol
Class IV	Slow calcium channel blockers	Verapamil, Diltiazem

The other important antiarrhythmic drugs (AADs) that are not in the Vaughan-Williams classification are digoxin and adenosine. Digoxin acts by inhibiting the Na/K pump, whereas adenosine acts on adenosine receptor.

The choice of drugs is dependent on many factors, such as nature of the AF, comorbidities, treatment strategy, clinical conditions of each patient, as well as patient preference. However, some general principles apply (Table 13.2).

Some of the antiarrhythmic drugs for AF would promote proarrhythmia (Table 13.3). Proarrhythmia is defined as the development of new arrhythmia or the worsening of the existing arrhythmia following antiarrhythmias initiation. It is best avoided by removing the precipitating factor.

Table 13.2 General principles on drugs for AF

Management strategy	Class of drugs
Paroxysmal AF and maintenance of sinus rhythm	Class Ia, Class Ic, Class II, Class III
Cardioversion	Class Ia, Class Ic, Class III
Rate control	Class II, Class III, Class IV, Digoxin

Table 13.3 Types of proarrhythmia during treatment with various antiarrhythmic drugs for AF or atrial flutter according to the Vaughan-Williams classification

Ventricular proarrhythmia

- Torsades de pointes (VW class Ia and III drugs)
- Sustained monomorphic ventricular tachycardia (usually VW class Ic drugs)
- Sustained polymorphic ventricular tachycardia/VF without long QT (VW class Ia, Ic, and III drugs)

Atrial proarrhythmia

- Provocation of recurrence (probably VW class Ia, Ic, and III drugs)
- Conversion of AF to flutter (usually VW class Ic drugs)
- Increase of defibrillation threshold (a potential problem with VW class Ic drugs)

Abnormalities of conduction or impulse formation

- Acceleration of ventricular rate during AF (VW class Ia and Ic drugs)
- Accelerated conduction over accessory pathway (digoxin, intravenous verapamil, or diltiazem)
- Sinus node dysfunction, atrioventricular block (almost all drugs)

VW = Vaughan-Williams classification
VF = ventricular fibrillation

General Non surgical Management Strategies

The overall management strategies for AF are based on rhythm control, rate control, and antithrombotic therapy. Patients with AF have to be assessed thoroughly, and their management should be guided by symptoms, whether there is any hemodynamic compromise or other associated comorbidities.[7] The above classification will help define the objectives of management and therapeutic strategies.

The main objective in the management of paroxysmal AF is to reduce paroxysmal event and maintain sinus rhythm, hence anti-arrhythmic drugs are used. Heart rate control is essential in patients with permanent AF, and hence, rate control drugs are used.

A rhythm control or rate control strategy can be used as first-line management in patients with persistent AF, and many patients will need both (Fig. 13.1).[6,7] All patients with AF have to be assessed on thromboembolic risk, and appropriate antithrombotic treatment is initiated.

Rate Control in Acute AF

After a thorough assessment of patients presenting with acute AF, the underlying causes and precipitating factors have to be identified and treated accordingly. If the patient becomes hemodynamically compromised due to the rapid ventricular rate, an emergency cardioversion should be employed (see later).

For patients who are hemodynamically stable, asymptomatic, or have presented >48 h of onset, a strategy of rate control and anticoagulation would leave sufficient time to determine the cause of AF.

In acute setting, we should probably aim for a resting heart rate of <100 beats/min, as suggested by the pooled analysis from Atrial Fibrillation Follow-up Investigation of Rhythm Management (AFFIRM) and Rate Control versus Electrical Cardioversion (RACE).[8] A well-controlled heart rate, which can be achieved by intravenous or oral use of atrioventricular (AV) nodal blocking drugs – for example verapamil, diltiazem, beta blockers and digoxin – would improve hemodynamic status and alleviate symptoms.

The rate-limiting calcium channel blockers (verapamil and diltiazem) are very effective in control heart rate during AF, and current management guidelines recommend these drug classes as first-line therapy for rate control. For a patient who has fast AF with mild left ventricle (LV) dysfunction or hypotension, diltiazem is the drug of choice, as it has less negative inotropic and peripheral vasodilatation effects compared to verapamil. Beta blockers are also effective rate control agents. Both groups of drugs have to be used with caution in patients with heart failure or hypotension.

Digoxin is often used in patients with fast AF and acute heart failure owing to its negative chronotropic and positive inotropic effects.[9] In hypotensive patients, digoxin is also an alternative to rate limiting calcium channel blockers and beta blockers – although the onset of action could take up to several hours. Digoxin is also not very effective in patients who are in high catecholamines state, such as postoperative, sepsis, myocardial ischemia, and pulmonary diseases.[9] Combination of digoxin with rate limiting calcium channel blockers and beta blockers might be needed to control ventricular rate, but a combination of verapamil and beta blockers should be avoided due to risk of ventricular asystole.

Amiodarone is a safe alternative if other drugs are ineffective or contraindicated in controlling ventricular rate, especially in patients with severe heart failure or hypotension. Intravenous amiodarone should be given via central venous line to prevent thrombophlebitis.

All patients in acute AF have to receive thromboprophylaxis therapy unless contraindicated. Unfractionated heparin or low molecular weight heparin should be used until a full assessment has been made and appropriate antithrombotic therapy has been commenced.[6]

Cardioversion in Acute AF

Patient presenting acutely with life-threatening hemodynamic stability should be treated with emergency electrical cardioversion, using heparin as antithrombotic cover. Both electrical and pharmacological cardioversion can safely be done on patients who do not have valvular heart disease and present with recent onset (less than 48 h) of AF using heparin (unfractionated or low molecular weight).

If the onset is more than 48 h or unclear, formal anticoagulation with an INR (International Normalization Ratio) of 2.0 or more is recommended for a minimum of 3 weeks before electrical cardioversion. Warfarin should be continued for a minimum of 4 weeks postcardioversion to prevent any thrombus formation due to atrial stunning in the postcardioversion period. For patients who are at high risk of thromboembolism or with any risk factors for recurrent AF, consideration should be given to lifelong anticoagulation.[6]

For centers or hospitals that are able to arrange a transesophageal echocardiogram (TEE), an immediate cardioversion can be performed once atrial thrombus has been ruled out (a TEE-guided cardioversion approach).

As discussed above, both Class I and Class III drugs can be used for pharmacological cardioversion. The success rate is variable depending on the duration of AF. AF of <48 h can be successfully cardioverted to sinus rhythm in 47–84% of patients within 24 h.[10] For AF that is longer in duration, the success rate is only 15–30%.[5,6] Class I drugs are contraindicated in patients who have structural heart disease due to the proarrhythmia risk. If pharmacological cardioversion fails, electrical cardioversion can still be attempted. There are studies that show that pretreatment with Class I and Class III drugs help facilitate electrical cardioversion and prevent recurrent atrial fibrillation.[5,6,11]

Despite antiarrhythmic drugs, approximately 50% of subjects relapse at 1 year. Factors that indicate high risk of AF recurrence include a history of failed cardioversion, structural heart disease, which includes mitral valve disease, left ventricular dysfunction, or enlarged left atrium, >12 months history of AF, and previous recurrences of AF.[5,6,12] Figure 13.2 summarizes the management of new onset of atrial fibrillation.

Paroxysmal AF

The main management objective in paroxysmal AF is the reduction of paroxysmal events and the long-term maintenance of sinus rhythm. Patients who have infrequent paroxysmal attacks or few symptoms, a "no drug treatment" strategy or "pill-in-the-pocket" strategy can be considered.[6,13] Those patients considered for a

Fig. 13.2 Management of new onset of atrial fibrillation

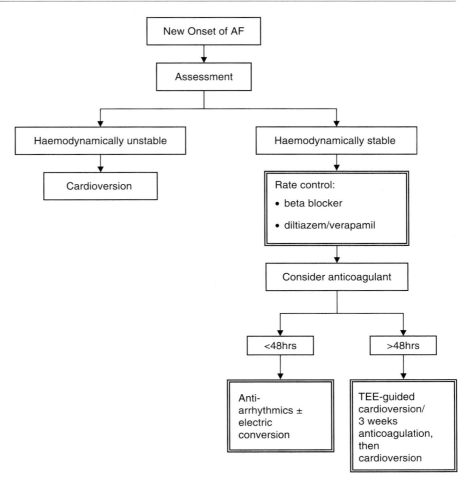

"pill-in-the-pocket" strategy should have no history of left ventricular dysfunction and valvular or ischemic heart disease and be able to understand how and when to take medication appropriately should a paroxysm occur.[13] Drugs that can be used in this strategy are Class 1c (flecainide, propafenone) and beta blockers. Figure 13.3 shows an algorithm for management of paroxysmal AF.

The initial treatment option for patients with frequent symptomatic paroxysmal AF (with or without structural heart disease, including coronary artery disease) is beta blockers. For patients who have no structural heart disease and where beta blockers are ineffective, a Class Ic agent or sotalol can be tried. If this approach still fails to provide adequate reduction in symptoms and paroxysms, either amiodarone or referral for nonpharmacological intervention (see later) should be considered. Class I drugs are contraindicated in patients who have structural heart disease due to the proarrhythmia risk. Digoxin should not be used in paroxysmal AF, as it has no effect on reduction in paroxysmal events. In fact, digoxin might make paroxysmal AF worse.

All patients should be assessed for thromboembolic risk and appropriate antithrombotic therapy should be initiated (see later).

Persistent AF

Patients with persistent AF can be treated either with rhythm control (Fig. 13.4) or rate control (Fig. 13.5) strategy. There are several clinical trials[14–17] comparing rhythm control with rate control for AF, and these consistently show that there is no significant difference

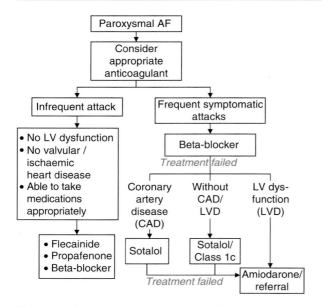

Fig. 13.3 Algorithm for the management of paroxysmal atrial fibrillation. LV=left ventricle

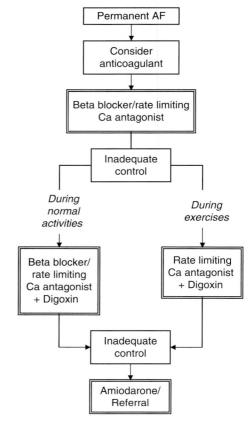

Fig. 13.5 Rate control treatment algorithm for permanent (and some cases of persistent) atrial fibrillation

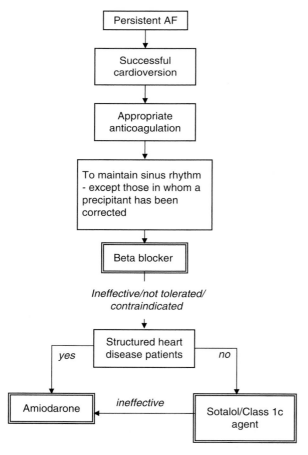

Fig. 13.4 Rhythm control algorithm for persistent atrial fibrillation

between the two strategies, that is, rate control is not an inferior strategy to a rhythm control one.[15] The choice of which strategy to adopt should take into account of any comorbidities, symptoms, and patient preferences.

The NICE guidelines[6] have suggested that a "rate control strategy" should be the preferred initial option for patients who are over 65 years old; those with coronary artery disease; patients with contraindications to antiarrhythmic drugs; those who are unsuitable for cardioversion; and patients without congestive heart failure. On the other hand, a "rhythm control strategy" should be the preferred initial option for patients who are symptomatic and younger; those presenting for the first time with lone AF; patients with congestive heart failure; and those with AF secondary to treated/corrected precipitant. Since publication of the NICE guidelines, a clinical trial in AF patients with congestive heart failure (CHF) has been presented (the AF-CHF trial[16]), showing that there was no significant difference between a rate control or rhythm control strategy in this patient group. In this trial ($n = 1,376$), which was a prospective, open-label, multicenter trial, AF patients with left ventricular ejection fraction (LVEF) of ≤35% and symptoms of CHF (NYHA class II–IV) were enrolled; asymptomatic patients could be enrolled, if they had a prior hospitalization for CHF or an LVEF <25%.

For patients who have opted for rhythm control strategy, either pharmacological or electrical cardioversion can be used. If AF is successfully cardioverted, beta blockers can be used to help maintain sinus rhythm. When beta blockers are ineffective, not tolerated, or contraindicated, or if the patient had previously relapsed to AF while on them, Class Ic agents can be tried provided the patient has no structural heart disease. If this drug fails or the patient has structural heart disease, amiodarone is the next option. If the patient fails to remain in sinus rhythm despite antiarrhythmic drugs to prevent relapse, then a rate control strategy should be adopted.

Patients who have opted for rate control strategy should be treated as permanent AF. Irrespective of which strategy is used, patients should be on appropriate antithrombotic therapy according to risk stratification (as discussed later).

Permanent AF

Patients who have AF for a long period of time, as well as those who have failed or are unsuitable for cardioversion should be treated with a rate control strategy. The ventricular rate in AF is generally considered to be "controlled" when the rate is 60–90 beats/min at rest and 90–115 beats/min during moderate exercise.[5] It has been suggested that AF patients should probably have a heart rate, which is faster than that which would be present if the patient was in sinus rhythm, to maintain an equivalent cardiac output.[17]

As discussed previously, a rate control strategy can be achieved by using pharmacological agents that act on the atrioventricular (AV) node. Drugs that are commonly used are beta blockers, rate-limiting calcium channel blockers, and digoxin. Digoxin is not very effective in controlling heart rate during exercise because of lack of vagal tone during activities. Thus, digoxin is only advised to be used as monotherapy for the elderly sedentary patient.

Both beta blockers and rate-limiting calcium channel blockers are effective as monotherapy for rate control. Some patients do need a combination of drugs to control ventricular rate.[18,19] When monotherapy is not adequate, beta blockers or rate-limiting calcium channel blockers should be given in combination with digoxin to control heart rate only during normal activities. If heart rate control is needed in both normal activities and exercise, rate-limiting calcium channel blockers should be given with digoxin.[6,20,21] Amiodarone can be used if further rate control is needed.

Nonpharmacological Treatments for AF

Antiarrhythmic drugs have limited efficacy and proarrhythmic risks. This has prompted the exploration of alternative nonpharmacological therapies to treat AF. Most of the nonpharmacological therapy approaches are directed to eliminate the triggers and to modify the electrophysiological substrate for the prevention and treatment for AF. In some patients, a combination of approaches (so-called "hybrid therapy") could be used for successful rhythm control.[22]

The recognition of the pulmonary vein as the common source of rapidly depolarizing arrhythmogenic foci that induces paroxysmal AF and the success in surgical approach (e.g., Maze procedure) have provided a platform for several ablation therapies. For patients with paroxysmal AF, elimination of these foci can achieve a success rate of as high as 90%.[23,24] Nonetheless, the success rate does depend on operator experience and the different techniques that are employed for the procedure. In specialized centers with extensive experience in AF ablation, the success of different catheter ablation techniques seems to be comparable (roughly 80%), especially if a tailored approach is used.[25]

In patients with conventional indications for pacemaker implantations (sinus node disease, symptomatic bradycardia, and chronotropic incompetence), dual-chamber or atrial pacemaker has been shown to prevent AF compared to single-chamber ventricular pacemakers.[26] The use of the implantable cardioverter defibrillator for primary or secondary prevention of ventricular arrhythmias could stop AF and reduce the burden of the arrhythmia; however, there is no role for the stand-alone atrial defibrillators in the treatment of AF.[27] The nonpharmacological therapies also come with some adverse effects (Table 13.4).

Table 13.4 Nonpharmacological (but nonsurgical) treatments for atrial fibrillation

	Current indications	Adverse effects
Device therapies		
Atrial pacing	Patients with conventional indications for pacemaker	Shock discomfort
Defibrillator	Patients with conventional indications for implantable cardioverter defibrillator	Early reinitiation of AF
AV nodal ablation and permanent pacing	Symptomatic patients refractory to other rate-control and rhythm-control treatments	Pacemaker dependence
	Patients who already have an implanted pacemaker or defibrillator	Sudden death early after ablation (<0.1%)
Catheter ablation	Symptomatic patients refractory to AADs	Vascular access complications (1%)
	Young patients with lone AF	Stroke and transient ischemic attack (1%)
	Patients unable or unwilling to take long-term AADs	Pronounced pulmonary vein stenosis (<1%)
		Proarrhythmia (10–20%)
		Rare: valvular, phrenic nerve, and esophagus injury

AV = atrio-ventricular; AADs = antiarrhythmic drugs

Antithrombotic Therapy

AF patients have increased risk of thromboembolic events. The risk of stroke or thromboembolism is four-fold to fivefold across all age groups, and is similar in patients with either paroxysmal or permanent AF.[28]

Irrespective of a rhythm control or rate control strategy, antithrombotic therapy is an essential part of AF management. Indeed, a rhythm control strategy does not necessarily reduce the risk of thromboembolism, and current guidelines even suggest that if the risk of recurrence AF is high, lifelong anticoagulation should be considered after cardioversion.[6] Patients with atrial flutter should be managed similarly to those patients with AF, depending on the coexistence of stroke risk factors.

Appropriate choice of thromboprophylaxis in AF is not an easy task, since the risk of stroke is not homogeneous among all AF subjects and treatment has to balance stroke risk, contraindications, and comorbidities.[6,29] High-risk factors include previous stroke or transient ischemic attack; age >75 years; presence of moderate to severe LV dysfunction; and those with structural heart disease, hypertension, diabetes mellitus, or vascular disease. Of all the various risk stratification schemes, CHADS2 (Congestive heart failure, Hypertension, Age>75, Diabetes, previous Stroke, or transient ischemic attack) is the most popular and well-validated scheme.[30]

A practical algorithm-based risk stratification scheme for thromboprophylaxis in AF is summarized in Fig. 13.6, as recommended by the UK NICE guidelines for AF management. The NICE guideline classifies patients into low-risk, moderate-risk, and high-risk groups. All AF patients should be assessed individually based on this scheme and should be treated accordingly.

One of the important risks for antithrombotic agents is bleeding. The assessment of bleeding risk becomes part of the clinical assessment of patients with AF before starting anticoagulation therapy. Risk factors associated with anticoagulation-related bleeding complications are broadly recognized and can include elderly age, uncontrolled hypertension, history of myocardial infarction or ischemic heart disease, cerebrovascular disease, anemia or history of bleeding, and the concomitant use of other medications such as antiplatelet agents.[31] The potential risks and benefits should always be explained to patients.

Future Perspectives

The role of renin-angiotensin-aldosterone system (RAAS) in AF has been reported quite extensively. RAAS blockade with angiotensin-converting enzyme inhibitors and angiotensin receptor blockers could play

Fig. 13.6 Stroke risk stratification algorithm. TIA = transient ischemic attack; LV = left ventricle

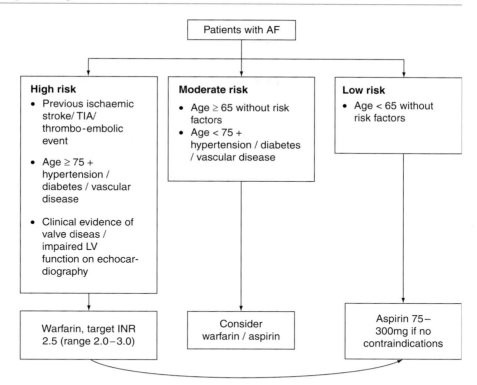

a role in prevention of AF and maintenance of sinus rhythm post cardioversion.[32,33] The role of inflammation has also been explored in AF, and inflammation may precede the development of AF, contribute to its persistence, and "drive" the prothrombotic state in AF.[34]

New antiarrhythmic drugs such as dronedarone may well change our approach to rhythm control, for cardioversion of AF and the maintenance of sinus rhythm.[35] Dronedarone is a noniodinated amiodarone-like drug that has more potent electrophysiological properties and less extracardiac toxicity than amiodarone. Some other new AADs, which are in development, would hopefully overcome some of the limitations of the existing agents.

Given the limitations of the vitamin K antagonists (e.g., warfarin) such as the substantial inter- and intrapatient variability in anticoagulation intensity, as monitored by the International Normalized Ratio, there is considerable interest in finding new oral anticoagulants that do not require monitoring and have few drug and food interactions. Two new drug classes, the oral direct thrombin inhibitors and oral factor Xa inhibitors, are promising alternatives to warfarin, and ongoing clinical trials in AF are still in progress.

Given the landscape would change with the availability of the new oral anticoagulants that overcome the dis-utility of warfarin, stroke risk stratification is likely to evolve, to enable more widespread use of oral anticoagulation.

Whilst the CHADS2 score is commonly used given its simplicity, it has many limitations, and does not include many stroke risk factors. To complement the CHADS2 score, a new risk factor based schema has been proposed, the CHA2DS2-VASc score (see table 13.5) [36]

When patients have a CHADS2 score of 2 or more, such patients clearly merit anticoagulation. where patients have a CHADS2 score or 0-1 or where a more comprehensive stroke risk assessment is needed, additional stroke risk modifiers should be considered, within the CHA2DS2-VASc score.

If so, those with a CHA2DS2-VASc score of 2 or more, oral anticoagulation is clearly recommended (whether with warfarin or the new oral anticoagulant agents). In those with a CHA2DS2-VASc score of 1, oral anticoagulation or antiplatelet therapy can be considered, but oral anticoagulant is preferred, given the marked benefits for oral anticoagulation over antiplatelet

Table 13.5 Score for assessing stroke risk (CHA$_2$DS$_2$-VASc) and Bleeding risk (HAS-BLED)

Letters	CHA$_2$DS$_2$-VASc	Score
C	Congestive heart failure/LV dysfunction	1
H	Hypertension	1
A	Aged ≥75 years	2
D	Diabetes mellitus	1
S	Stroke/TIA/TE	2
V	Vascular disease [prior MI, PAD, or aortic plaque]	1
A	Aged 65-74 years	1
S	Sex category [i.e. female gender]	1
Maximun Score		9
Letters	Clinical characteristic [a]	Score
C	Hypertension	1
A	Abnormal renal and liver function (1 point each)	1 or 2
S	Stroke	1
B	Bleeding	1
L	Labile INRs	1
E	Elderly	1
D	Drugs or alcohol (1 point each)	1 or 2
Maximun Score		9

[a] 'Hypertension' is defined as systolic blood pressure >160 mmHg. 'Abnormal renal function' is defined as the presence of chronic dialysis or renal transplantation or serum creatinine ≥200 μmol/L. 'Abnormal liver function' is defined as chronic hepatic disease (e.g., cirrhosis) or biochemical evidence of significant hepatic derangement (eg. bilirubin >2x upper limit of normal, in association with AST/ALT/ALP >3x upper limit normal, etc). 'Bleeding' refers to previous bleeding history and/or predisposition to bleeding e.g. bleeding diathesis, anemia, etc. 'Labile INRs' refers to unstable/high INRs or poor time in therapeutic range (eg. <60%). Drugs/alcohol use refers to concomitant use of drugs, such as anti-platelet agents, non-steroidal anti-inflammatory drugs, etc

therapy in this patient group. Patients with a CHA2DS2-VASc score = 0, such patients are 'truly low risk' and no antithrombotic therapy or aspirin can be used, with preference for no antithrombotic therapy, given the lack of benefit for aspirin in low risk AF patients, and the potential for harm, with bleeding.

New bleeding risk scoring assessments, such as the HAS-BLED scheme, would also assist management by helping clinicians assess bleeding risk with a simple, user-friendly scoring system [37] (Table 13.5).

Conclusion

Patients presenting with atrial fibrillation should be assessed carefully and thoroughly. All precipitating causes should be treated. The choices of treatment on the irregular rhythm itself are individually based. Both rhythm control and rate control therapy can be employed as first-line treatment, depending on the duration of irregular rhythm. General principles on drugs for treatment of atrial fibrillation are listed in Table 13.2. All patients present with atrial fibrillation should also be assessed on thromboembolic risks, and appropriate antithrombotic therapy should be started.

References

1. Lloyd-Jones DM, Wang TJ, Leip EP, et al. Lifetime risk for development of atrial fibrillation: the Framingham heart study. *Circulation*. 2004;110:1042-1046.
2. Fox CS, Parise H, D'Agostino RB Sr, et al. Parental atrial fibrillation as a risk factor for atrial fibrillation in offspring. *JAMA*. 2004;291:2851-2855.
3. Waldo AL. Mechanism of atrial fibrillation. *J Cardiovasc Electrophysiol*. 2003;14(12 Suppl): S267-S274.
4. Saffitz JE. Connexins, conduction, and atrial fibrillation. *N Engl J Med*. 2006;354(25):2712-2714.
5. Watson T, Shantsila E, Lip GYH. Mechanisms of thrombogenesis in atrial fibrillation. Virchow's triad revisited. Lancet 2008;372.
6. National Collaborating Centre for Chronic Conditions. Atrial Fibrillation: national clinical guideline for management in primary and secondary care. London: Royal College of Physicians, 2006 (http://rcplondon.ac.uk/pubs/books/af/index.asp).
7. Lip GY, Tse HF. Management of atrial fibrillation. *Lancet*. 2007;370:604-618.
8. Van Gelder IC, Wyse DG, Chandler ML, Cooper HA, Olshansky B, Hagens VE, Crijns HJ, RACE and AFFIRM. Does intensity of rate-control influence outcome in artial fribrillation. An analysis of pooled date from the RACE and AFFIRM studies. *Europace*. 2006; 8:935–942.
9. Li Saw Hee FL, Lip GYH. Digoxin revisited. *QJM*. 1998; 91:259-264.
10. Naccarelli GV, Wolbrette DL, Khan M, et al. Old and new antiarrythmic drugs for converting and maintaining sinus rhythm in atrial fibrillation: comparative efficacy and results of trials. *Am J Cardiol*. 2003;91:15-26D.
11. Singh BN, Singh SN, Reda DJ, Tang XC, Lopez B, Harris CL, Fletcher RD, Sharma SC, Atwood JE, Jacobson AK, Lewis HD Jr, Raisch DW, Ezekowitz MD, Sotalol Amiodarone Atrial Fibrillation Efficacy Trial (SAFE-T) Investigators. Amiodarone versus sotalol for atrial fibrillation. *N Engl J Med*. 2005;352:1861-1872.

12. Singer DE, Albers GW, Dalen JE, et al. Antithrombotic therapy in atrial fibrillation: American College of Chest Physicians Evidence-Based Clinical Practice Guidelines (8th Edition). *Chest*. 2008;133(6 Suppl):546S-592S.

13. Alboni P, Botto GL, Baldi N, et al. Outpatient treatment of recent-onset atrial fibrillation with the "pill-in-the-pocket" approach. *N Engl J Med*. 2004;351:2384-2391.

14. Hohnloser SH, Kuck KH, Lilienthal J. Rhythm or rate control in atrial fibrillation – pharmacological intervention in atrial fibrillation (PIAF): a randomised trial. *Lancet*. 2000; 356:1789-1794.

15. Testa L, Biondi-Zoccai GG, Dello Russo A, Bellocci F, Andreotti F, Crea F. Rate-control vs. rhythm-control in patients with atrial fibrillation: a meta-analysis. *Eur Heart J*. 2005;26(19):2000-2006.

16. Roy D, Talajic M, Nattel S, et al. Rhythm control versus rate control for atrial fibrillation and heart failure. *N Engl J Med*. 2008;358(25):2667-2677.

17. Rawles JM. What is meant by a 'controlled' ventricular rate in atrial fibrillation? *Br Heart J*. 1990;63:157-161.

18. Khand AU, Rankin AC, Martin W, Taylor J, Gemmell I, Cleland JG. Carverdilol alone or in combination with digoxin for the management of atrial fibrillation in patients with heart failure? *J Am Coll Cardiol*. 2003;42:1944-1951.

19. Segal JB, McNamara RL, Miller MR, et al. The evidence regarding the drugs used for ventricular rate control. *J Fam Pract*. 2000;49:47-59.

20. Farshi R, Kistner D, Sarma JS, Longmate JA, Singh BN. Ventricular rate control in chronic atrial fibrillation during daily activity and programmed exercise: a crossover open label study of five drug regimens. *J Am Coll Cardiol*. 1999; 33:304-310.

21. Roth A, Harrison E, Mitani G, Cohen J, Rahimtoola SH, Elkayam U. Efficacy and safety of medium-and high-dose diltiazem alone and in combination with digoxin for control of heart rate at rest and during exercise in patients with chronic atrial fibrillation. *Circulation*. 1986;73:316-324.

22. Saksena S, Madan N. Hybrid therapy of atrial fibrillation: algorithms and outcome. *J Interv Card Electriohysiol*. 2003;9:235-247.

23. Oral H, Knight BP, Tada H, et al. Pulmonary vein isolation for paroxysmal and persistent atrial fibrillation. *Circulation*. 2002;105:1077-1081.

24. Marrouche NF, Martin DO, Wazni O, et al. Phased-array intracardiac echocardiography monitoring during pulmonary vein isolation in patients with atrial fibrillation: impact on outome and complications. *Circulation*. 2003; 107: 2710-2716.

25. Oral H, Chugh A, Good E, et al. A tailored approach to catheter ablation of paroxysmal atrial fibrillation. *Circulation*. 2006;113:1824-1831.

26. Healey JS, Toff WD, Lamas GA, et al. Cardiovascular outcomes with atrial-based pacing compared with ventricular pacing: meta-analysis of randomized trials, using individual patient data. *Circulation*. 2006;114:11-17.

27. Friedman PA, Dijkman B, Warman EN, et al. Atrial therapies reduce atrial arrhythmia burden in defibrillator patients. *Circulation*. 2001;104:1023-1028.

28. Lip GY, Boss CJ. Antithrombotic treatment in atrial fibrillation. *Heart*. 2006;92:155-161.

29. Hughes M, Lip GY, Guideline Development Group, National Clinical Guideline for Management of Atrial Fibrillation in Primary and Secondary Care, National Institute for Health and Clinical Excellence. Stroke and thromboembolism in atrial fibrillation: a systematic review of stroke risk factors, risk stratification schema and cost effectiveness data. *Thromb Haemost*. 2008;99(2):295-304.

30. Gage BF, van Walraven C, Pearce L, et al. Selecting patients with atrial fibrillation for anticoagulation: stroke risk stratification in patients taking aspirin. *Circulation*. 2004;110: 2287-2292.

31. Hughes M, Lip GY, on behalf of the Guideline Development Group for the NICE national clinical guideline for management of atrial fibrillation in primary and secondary care. Risk factors for anticoagulation-related bleeding complications in patients with atrial fibrillation: a systematic review. *QJM*. 2007;100:599-607.

32. Healey JS, Baranchuk A, Crystal E, et al. Prevention of atrial fibrillation with angiotensin-converting enzyme inhibitors and angiotensin receptor blockers: a meta-analysis. *J Am Coll Cardiol*. 2005;45:1832-1839.

33. Boos CJ, Lip GY. Targeting the renin-angiotensin-aldosterone system in atrial fibrillation: from pathophysiology to clinical trials. *J Hum Hypertens*. 2005;19:855-859.

34. Boos CJ, Anderson R, Lip GYH. Is atrial fibrillation an inflammatory disorder? *Eur Heart J*. 2006;27:136-149.

35. Stiles S. Dronedarone safety, efficacy standings bolstered in huge atrial-fibrillation trial. theheart.org. [HeartWire > Electrophysiology]; May 19, 2008. Available at: http://www.theheart.org/article/867591.do. Accessed June 24, 2008.

36. Lip GY, Nieuwlaat R, Pisters R, et al. Refining clinical risk stratification for predicting stroke and thromboembolism in atrial fibrillation using a novel risk factor-based approach: the Euro Heart Survey on atrial fibrillation. Chest, 2010; 137, 263-272.

37. Pisters R, Lane DA, Nieuwlaat R, et al. A novel user-friendly score (HAS-BLED) to assess one-year risk of major bleeding in atrial fibrillation patients: The Euro Heart Survey. Chest 2010;Mar 18.[Epub]. doi: 10.1378/chest.10-134.

Ablation of Atrial Fibrillation with Cardiac Surgery

14

Adam E. Saltman and A. Marc Gillinov

Introduction

Atrial fibrillation (AF) is common in patients presenting for mitral valve surgery. Routine ablation of AF in such patients, although still not applied universally, is a recent phenomenon. This may be attributable to new data clarifying the pathogenesis of AF, the dangers of leaving it untreated, and development of new technologies that facilitate ablation. With a more comprehensive approach toward treating both the arrhythmia and the structural heart disease, it is estimated that surgeons could perform more than 10,000 ablation procedures annually. The purposes of this review are to (1) present the rationale for surgical ablation of AF in mitral valve patients, (2) describe the classic Maze procedure and its results, (3) detail new approaches to surgical ablation of AF, (4) emphasize the importance of the left atrial appendage, and (5) consider challenges and future directions in the ablation of AF in cardiac surgical patients.

Rationale for Surgical Ablation

AF Prevalence

AF is present in up to 50% of patients undergoing mitral valve surgery[1-3], and therefore, most studies examining concomitant ablation focus on this group.

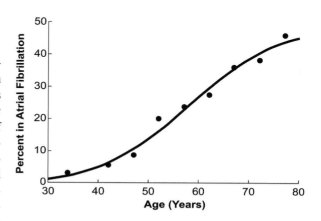

Fig. 14.1 Prevalence of atrial fibrillation versus age in patients with degenerative mitral valve disease

As in the general population, the prevalence of AF in patients with mitral valve disease increases with patient age (Fig. 14.1). Patients with AF also have a worse New York Heart Association functional class, more severe left ventricular dysfunction, and greater left atrial enlargement.[4-6] Recently published data examining patients undergoing coronary artery bypass grafting (CABG) confirms similar associations of AF in this population.[7]

AF Dangers

AF is associated with increased mortality and morbidity in mitral valve and CABG patients,[3,7,8] as well as in those not undergoing surgery.[3] If left untreated at the time of valve replacement or repair, AF is unlikely to resolve[4-6,9] and its ongoing presence is both a marker and a risk factor for increased late mortality.[10] In addition, the presence of AF is associated with stroke,

A.E. Saltman (✉)
Atrial Fibrillation Center and Cardiothoracic Surgery Research, Department of Cardiothoracic Surgery, Maimonides Medical Center, Brooklyn, New York, USA
e-mail: adamsaltman@gmail.com

R.S. Bonser et al. (eds.), *Mitral Valve Surgery*,
DOI: 10.1007/978-1-84996-426-5_14, © Springer-Verlag London Limited 2011

peripheral thromboembolism, anticoagulant-related hemorrhage, symptomatic tachycardia, reduced cardiac output, and tachycardia-induced cardiomyopathy.[8–12] This is particularly deleterious in patients with structural heart disease and reduced cardiac output. For these reasons, the concomitant treatment of AF is strongly recommended when formulating an operative strategy for patients with mitral valve disease.

AF Mechanisms and Implications for Surgical Ablation

Over the past decade, the treatment of AF has varied widely from the classical approach described by Cox: wide encirclement of the pulmonary veins, ablation to the mitral annulus, additional lesions in the right atrium, and amputation of the atrial appendages.[13] There are now published multiple series of patients undergoing simple pulmonary vein ablation, posterior left atrial isolation, and poorly described "modified maze" procedures, all for different indications and all with different devices and techniques. Such a confusion has made the comparison difficult.

Furthermore, because the pathogenesis of AF in cardiac surgical patients is incompletely understood, and probably varies among individuals, there is no consensus concerning what specific ablation strategy should be used for which patients. Recognition of this phenomenon has engendered different AF classification schemes such as "paroxysmal," "persistent," or "permanent"[14] or even "intermittent" or "continuous"[15]; however, the extent to which the different mechanisms of focal activity and/or re-entry contribute to the initiation and maintenance of AF remains disputed.[16] Yet while the electrophysiologic causes of AF await further investigation, the anatomical basis of AF is becoming increasingly clear.

In patients with isolated AF, endocardial electrophysiologic mapping data have shown that the pulmonary veins and posterior left atrium are critical anatomic sites for most patients,[17,18] although the superior vena cava and left atrial appendage may also contribute in some.[19–21] Unfortunately, because intraoperative mapping in individual cardiac surgical patients is time-consuming and technically demanding, especially when concomitant procedures are being performed,

there is less evidence supporting this concept in patients with mitral valve disease. Nevertheless, the available studies do support the importance of the left atrium as the most common driving chamber: rapid and repetitive activation can be identified in the posterior left atrium around the pulmonary vein orifices and left atrial appendage in many patients.[22–26] The right atrium may play a lesser role.[22]

Although some attempts are being made to tailor the ablative approach to surgical patients on the basis of real-time intraoperative mapping,[27] such a technology is not routinely available. Therefore, an anatomic approach to ablation based on our understanding of pathophysiology and empiric results is still reasonable. A left atrial-based procedure that includes an encircling lesion around all four pulmonary veins with a lesion to the mitral annulus eliminates AF in 70–90% of mitral valve patients.[26,28–31] The addition of right atrial lesions in these patients is controversial.[32,33] On the one hand, it may increase the rate of cure,[33,34] but on the other, it may increase the risk for typical atrial flutter.[35] However, right atrial lesion creation is simple and does not appreciably increase operative time; any resulting flutter is easily treated percutaneously. Therefore, AF ablation in mitral valve patients should probably entail treatment of both atria.

The Maze Procedure

The Cox Maze III operation, or Maze procedure, has a 20-year history and is the most effective curative therapy for AF yet devised.[36–39] It is the gold standard for surgical treatment of AF and newer approaches and techniques must be measured against it.

In the Maze procedure, multiple left and right atrial incisions and cryolesions are placed to interrupt the multiple reentrant circuits of AF (Fig. 14.2). The Maze lesions include isolation of the pulmonary veins and posterior left atrium and excision of the left atrial appendage; these maneuvers are critical to the restoration of sinus rhythm and the reduction of the risk of thromboembolism.[40]

Although the Maze procedure is a complex operation that requires 45–60 min of cardiopulmonary bypass and cardiac arrest, experienced surgeons have performed the classic operation safely in large numbers of patients having concomitant cardiac surgery.[1,2,37,38] The

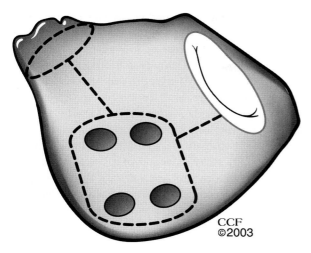

Fig. 14.2 Left atrial lesion set of the Maze procedure. *Small circles* represent pulmonary vein orifices and white oval represents the mitral valve. *Dashed lines* represent surgical incisions (Reprinted with permission, Cleveland Clinic Center for Medical Art & Photography © 2003-2010. All Rights Reserved)

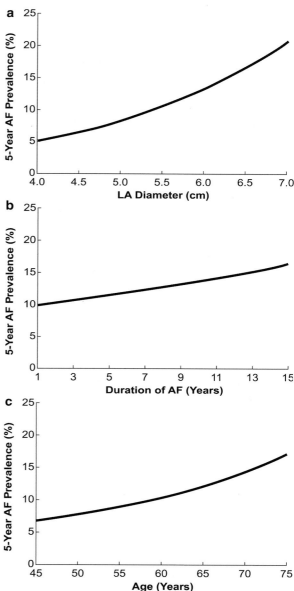

Fig. 14.3 Prevalence at 5 years of postoperative AF in patients having combined mitral valve surgery and a Maze procedure demonstrating effects of selected preoperative factors. (**a**) Left atrial (LA) diameter. (**b**) Preoperative duration of AF. (**c**) Age (From Prasad et al.[39] Used with permission)

addition of a Maze procedure does not appear to increase operative mortality or morbidity.[39,41,42] However, it is associated with a 5–10% need for implantation of a permanent pacemaker, most commonly in those with pre-existing sinus node dysfunction or in patients having multivalve surgery. Recent data demonstrate that the Maze procedure has equivalent long-term efficacy in patients undergoing both lone operations and concomitant procedures.[39] Results of a concomitant Maze procedure vary somewhat between different groups; successful restoration of sinus rhythm has been achieved in 70–96% of patients.[39,41–43]

Early postoperative AF is common after the Maze procedure, usually abating by 3 months. However, over time, some patients develop recurrent AF.[39,41,42] The pathogenesis of this is unclear, but risk factors have been identified (Fig. 14.3). Increasing left atrial diameter, longer duration of preoperative AF, and advanced patient age all increase the late prevalence of AF.[44] Thus, 5 years after a concomitant Maze procedure, the predicted prevalence of AF is only 5% in mitral valve patients with a 4-cm left atrium; in contrast, the predicted prevalence is 15% in similar patients with a 6-cm left atrium. Others have identified similar risk factors for AF after the Maze procedure, suggesting the possibility that earlier operation and left atrial size reduction in those with left atrial enlargement (>6 cm) might improve results.[44–47]

Interestingly, the presenting pattern of AF (paroxysmal, persistent, or permanent) does not appear to impact the results of the Maze procedure.[42] Similarly, in mitral valve patients, the etiology of valve dysfunction does not influence results, and there is general agreement that the Maze procedure is effective in patients with rheumatic valve disease, as well as in those with degenerative mitral valve disease.[48,49] Even in patients with rheumatic disease, biatrial contraction is usually restored to some degree.[48,50]

The Maze procedure is associated with important clinical benefits beyond rhythm restoration in patients with mitral valve disease. Recent data demonstrate that restoration of sinus rhythm improves survival in these patients[10] and reduces the risk of stroke, other thromboembolism, and anticoagulant-related hemorrhage.[10–12,40]

The reduced risk of late stroke after a Maze procedure deserves particular emphasis. In the largest series focusing on this outcome, Cox noted only a single late stroke at a mean follow-up of 5 years in 300 patients having a classic Maze procedure.[40] This remarkable freedom from late stroke may be attributable to restoration of sinus rhythm, but more likely results from removal of the left atrial appendage, which is an integral component of the Maze procedure. This important maneuver will be discussed next.

Despite these excellent results, the Maze procedure has been relatively underutilized, and today the classical operation is almost obsolete. Indeed, as many mitral valve patients today present at a more advanced age and with more comorbidities, surgeons hesitate to add a classical Maze procedure and instead are turning to "less invasive," simpler techniques, often based on new ablation technologies. As this trend will likely continue, it becomes critical for the surgeon to understand the benefits and limitations of the various ablation strategies and tools.

New Approaches to Surgical Ablation of Atrial Fibrillation

Lesion Sets

Surgical techniques for AF ablation remain anatomically focused, concentrating on creation of lines of conduction block in the left atrium.[51–53] Because the left atrium is opened for mitral valve procedures, precise creation of lesions is possible from the endocardial aspect. A variety of lesion sets have been employed to ablate AF in patients with mitral valve disease. Most include pulmonary vein isolation, excision or exclusion

of the left atrial appendage, and linear left atrial connecting lesions.[51–55] The pulmonary veins may be isolated with a single box-like lesion or with separate right- and left-sided ovals around the pulmonary veins. With the advantage of direct vision, the surgeon can easily create a lesion from the left pulmonary veins to the mitral annulus; this lesion improves results, particularly in patients with permanent AF and mitral valve disease.[41,56–58] In patients with left atrial enlargement (>6 cm), left atrial reduction may also increase the chances of sinus rhythm restoration.[45]

The issue concerning the creation of bi-atrial lesions (more closely mimicking the traditional Maze set) versus creating left atrial lesions alone remains contentious. It is clearly easier and faster to create a more limited lesion set; yet recent data indicate that patients undergoing both right and left atrial treatment have a better long-term result at maintaining sinus rhythm.[33] Through the judicious selection of a technology or multiple technologies, as discussed later, it is now becoming possible to create right-sided lesions without opening the right atrium, prolonging cardiopulmonary bypass time or aortic cross-clamp time. In this manner, the largest number of patients can be treated in the most efficacious and safest fashion.

A Review of the Available Energy Sources

The classical lesion creation method is cutting and sewing tissue. This produces a transmural scar that is not electrically conductive. The goal of any energy source, therefore, is to create a similar scar by exposing tissue to extremes of temperature, inducing thermal injury, coagulation necrosis, and healing.

To produce such an injury, the tissue must be either heated to 50°C or frozen to −60°C.[59,60] The quantity of tissue injured is usually directly proportional to the duration of time for which the tissue is held at either temperature. The various energy sources discussed later differ mainly in the method by which they transfer energy to the tissue and how deeply that energy is conducted into the tissue. A summary review of some characteristics, advantages, and disadvantages of each method is given in Table 14.1.

Despite clearly different energy forms and application methods, it is interesting to note that when applied with the left atrium open, from the endocardial

Table 14.1 Characteristics, advantages, and disadvantages of methods of tissue ablation

Energy source	Method	Advantages	Disadvantages	Brand name
Dry unipolar RF	Contact resistive heating	1. Well-understood technology 2. High tissue temperatures achieved 3. Flexible delivery system	1. Poor temperature control 2. Fat does not heat well or conduct well 3. No transmurality feedback 4. Dosimetric energy delivery 5. Collateral damage from conduction into surrounding structures	Boston Scientific Cobra®
Irrigated unipolar RF	Contact resistive heating	1. Higher energy delivery at lower operating temperature 2. Small tip can make many lesions 3. Complete operator control over lesion set	1. Highly operator-dependent (Otherwise same as dry unipolar RF)	Medtronic Cardioblate®
Dry bipolar RF	Contact resistive heating	1. Shielded energy source 2. Very localized lesion 3. Possible transmurality feedback, used to control energy delivery 4. Very fast ablation times	1. Fixed device shape, limiting lesion types 2. Large device, making minimal access difficult	Atricure®
Irrigated bipolar RF	Contact resistive heating	1. Device more malleable than dry bipolar RF 2. Irrigation avoids char Otherwise as with dry bipolar RF	Same as dry bipolar RF (except more flexible delivery system)	Medtronic Cardioblate® BP
Hi-intensity focused ultrasound	Radiation into tissue	Penetrates fat well Does not require intimate tissue contact Shielded energy source Highly effective against heat "sink" of flowing blood	1. Difficult to control energy application 2. Rigid transducers make minimal access difficult	St. Judes Medical Epicor™
Laser	Radiation into tissue	1. Malleable device permits minimal access 2. Otherwise same as above, except not as effective against blood "sink"	1. Difficult to achieve full tissue penetration with flowing blood as energy "sink" 2. AtriLaze® wand is highly user-dependent	MedicalCV AtrilLaze® and SOLAR®
Cryothermy	Direct tissue freezing	1. Wide safety margin (Otherwise as with microwave)	1. Question about energy "sink" problems, Otherwise similar to microwave	Cooper Medical Frigitronics®; CryoCath SurgiFrost™

aspect with full cold cardioplegic arrest, there seems to be very little difference in the safety or efficacy of any one device over the others.[61] The first device used in treating AF during mitral valve surgery, and therefore the one with the largest published experience, is the dry unipolar radiofrequency (RF) Cobra® probe. The probe consists of a malleable 6 cm long × 2 mm diameter active tip that can be shaped as the operator desires. Surveying its reported use in 16 studies including 1,187 patients, Khargi and his colleagues found that dry unipolar RF was effective at freeing patients from AF 78% of the time (reported success ranged from 42% to 92%).[61] There have been several complications attributed to the use of the probe, however; the most worrisome were esophageal injuries, resulting in death 60% of the time.[62,63]

Of course, adverse events can occur with any technology when incorrectly applied,[64] but as more experience has been gained and safer methods of ablation have been developed, such as placing a cold, wet sponge between the posterior wall of the left atrium and the esophagus and/or shielding the probe in nonconducting sheaths, these injuries have become an extreme rarity.

The Left Atrial Appendage

Because 60–90% of stroke-causing emboli in AF patients originate from the left atrial appendage (LAA), this structure has been termed "our most lethal human attachment."[65] Therefore, excision or exclusion of the LAA is a critical component of operations to treat AF; this may explain in part the exceedingly low risk of stroke after the Maze procedure cited above. In fact, ligation of the LAA in mitral valve patients with AF reduces the late risk of thromboembolic events even if the patient does not have intraoperative ablation.[66]

It is essential for the surgeon to realize that the technique employed significantly impacts the results of LAA ligation, with incomplete ligation increasing the risk of thromboembolism.[67,68] Currently employed techniques include exclusion by suture ligation or noncutting stapler and excision with suture closure or stapling.[69] We currently favor surgical excision of the appendage with standard cut-and-sew techniques. Development of devices designed specifically for management of the LAA will hopefully facilitate this procedure both in speed and safety. Published preclinical experiences with new LAA occlusion devices are promising, and clinical trials are anticipated in the near future.[68,70]

Challenges and Future Directions

The variations in disease definitions, procedural details, and follow-up methods and treatments have significantly confounded our ability to further ablative therapy for patients with AF and mitral valve disease. Advances necessary to improve AF ablation in cardiac surgical patients include uniform definitions and methodology for reporting results, improved technology to facilitate ablation and its intraoperative assessment,

and refinement of minimally invasive procedures. Newer multidisciplinary reporting guidelines will help greatly toward clarifying the situation.[71]

Reporting Results

Standard terminology and methodology for reporting results is absent from the cardiac surgery and electrophysiology literature, and current reporting is haphazard and subject to criticism.[69] While there are now guidelines for categorizing the clinical pattern of AF (paroxysmal, persistent, or permanent), these are inconsistently applied. Techniques for postablation rhythm assessment vary, with no generally accepted standard. Ideally, simple and convenient technology for long-term and continuous rhythm monitoring will be developed. Data obtained with such systems could be analyzed in uniform fashions to determine (1) absolute freedom from AF, (2) AF burden in individual patients, and (3) prevalence of AF in treated populations.[4–6]

Ablation Technology and Intraoperative Assessment

Current surgical ablation technology has several limitations. No single ablation device enables creation of all lesions with ease of use, absence of collateral damage, and guaranteed lesion transmurality. In addition, because we do not yet have the capability to perform real-time mapping in the operating room, particularly if the heart is arrested, we cannot tailor an ablation procedure to a patient's particular electrophysiologic characteristics. Although anatomically based approaches are fairly successful, if we are to achieve anything close to a 100% cure rate, it is likely that a strategy based on both anatomic and electrophysiologic findings will be required.

Minimally Invasive Approaches

While most operations that include both mitral valve surgery and ablation are performed through a sternotomy, it is now possible to perform less invasive procedures quite safely and effectively. This may be achieved via a small right thoracotomy[72] or through a partial upper sternotomy. These procedures have been performed with bipolar radiofrequency, microwave, unipolar heat-based systems, and cryothermy.[72–74] However, they remain technically challenging. Minimally invasive or keyhole approaches using current technology are hampered by difficult access to the posterior left atrium and left atrial appendage, key targets for AF ablation. Further refinement in ablation technology is necessary to facilitate widespread application of minimally invasive cardiac surgery with ablation.

Conclusions

AF is common in patients presenting for cardiac surgery. Left untreated, AF increases morbidity and jeopardizes survival. Recent data demonstrate that AF ablation improves outcomes in these patients. Therefore, virtually all cardiac surgery patients with AF should have AF ablation, particularly those with mitral valve disease. The traditional cut-and-sew Maze procedure has become obsolete, replaced by operations that use alternate energy sources to create lines of conduction block rapidly with little risk of bleeding. Minimally invasive cardiac surgery with AF ablation is now possible. Continued progress will facilitate tailored ablation approaches for individual patients and further improve results.

Acknowledgments Data presented from The Cleveland Clinic Foundation were drawn from the experience of all staff surgeons and were collected by Kathleen M. Hill, R.N., and analyzed by Eugene H. Blackstone, M.D., and Jeevanantham Rajeswaran, M.Sc. New statistical methodology to assess success of ablation was developed by Dr. Blackstone and Mr. Rajeswaran. We thank Tess Knerik for her expert editorial assistance.

Disclosures Dr. Gillinov is a consultant to Edwards Lifesciences, LLC, Medtronic, Inc, and St. Jude Medical, Inc. He receives research support from the Atrial Fibrillation Innovation Center, a Third Frontier project funded by the State of Ohio and from the National Institutes of Health through Cleveland Clinic participation in the Cardiac Surgery Clinical Trials Network. The Cleveland Clinic has an indirect equity interest in AtriCure, Inc through its interest in a fund that has an equity interest in AtriCure, Inc.

Dr. Saltman is a consultant to and has received honoraria for speaking from Boston Scientific/Guidant Cardiac Surgery. He has received research support from Guidant, Medical CV and Estech LICS.

References

1. Cox JL. Intraoperative options for treating atrial fibrillation associated with mitral valve disease. *J Thorac Cardiovasc Surg*. 2001;122:212-215.
2. Ad N, Cox JL. Combined mitral valve surgery and the Maze III procedure. *Semin Thorac Cardiovasc Surg*. 2002;14: 206-209.
3. Grigioni F, Avierinos JF, Ling LH. Atrial fibrillation complicating the course of degenerative mitral regurgitation: determinants and long-term outcome. *J Am Coll Cardiol*. 2002; 40:84-92.
4. Obadia JF, el Farra M, Bastien OH. Outcome of atrial fibrillation after mitral valve repair. *J Thorac Cardiovasc Surg*. 1997;114:179-185.
5. Chua YL, Schaff HV, Orsulak TA. Outcome of mitral valve repair in patients with preoperative atrial fibrillation. Should the maze procedure be combined with mitral valvuloplasty? *J Thorac Cardiovasc Surg*. 1994;107:408-415.
6. Lim E, Barlow CW, Hosseinpour AR. Influence of atrial fibrillation on outcome following mitral valve repair. *Circulation*. 2001;104:I-59-I-63.
7. Quader MA, McCarthy PM, Gillinov AM, et al. Does preoperative atrial fibrillation reduce survival after coronary artery bypass grafting? *Ann Thorac Surg*. 2004; 77: 1514-1522.
8. Jessurun ER, van Hemel NM, Kelder JC. Mitral valve surgery and atrial fibrillation: is atrial fibrillation surgery also needed? *Eur J Cardiothorac Surg*. 2000;17:530-537.
9. Kalil RA, Maratia CB, D'Avila A. Predictive factors for persistence of atrial fibrillation after mitral valve operation. *Ann Thorac Surg*. 1999;67:614-617.
10. Bando K, Kasegawa H, Okada Y. The impact of pre- and postoperative atrial fibrillation on outcome after mitral valvuloplasty for nonischemic mitral regurgitation. *J Thorac Cardiovasc Surg*. 2005;129:1032-1040.
11. Bando K, Kobayashi J, Kosakai Y. Impact of Cox maze procedure on outcome in patients with atrial fibrillation and mitral valve disease. *J Thorac Cardiovasc Surg*. 2002;124: 575-583.
12. Handa N, Schaff HV, Morris JJ. Outcome of valve repair and the Cox maze procedure for mitral regurgitation and associated atrial fibrillation. *J Thorac Cardiovasc Surg*. 1999; 118: 628-635.
13. Cox JL. The surgical treatment of atrial fibrillation. IV. Surgical technique. *J Thorac Cardiovasc Surg*. 1991; 101(4): 584-592.
14. Fuster V, Ryden LE, Asinger RW, et al. ACC/AHA/ESC guidelines for the management of patients with atrial fibrillation. A report of the American College of Cardiology/American Heart Association Task Force on Practice Guidelines and the European Society of Cardiology Committee for Practice Guidelines and Policy Conferences (Committee to develop guidelines for the management of patients with atrial fibrillation) developed in collaboration with the North American Society of Pacing and Electrophysiology. *Eur Heart J*. 2001; 22(20): 1852-1923.
15. Cox JL. Atrial fibrillation I: a new classification system. *J Thorac Cardiovasc Surg*. 2003;126(6):1686-1692.

16. Wu T-J, Kerwin WF, Hwang C. Atrial fibrillation: focal activity, re-entry, or both? *Heart Rhythm.* 2004;1:117-120.

17. Haissaguerre M, Jais P, Shah DC, et al. Spontaneous initiation of atrial fibrillation by ectopic beats originating in the pulmonary veins. *N Engl J Med.* 1998;339:659-666.

18. Todd DM, Skanes AC, Guiraudon G, et al. Role of the posterior left atrium and pulmonary veins in human lone atrial fibrillation: electrophysiological and pathological data from patients undergoing atrial fibrillation surgery. *Circulation.* 2003;108(25):3108-3114.

19. Lee S-H, Tai C-T, Hsieh M-H, et al. Predictors of non-pulmonary vein ectopic beats initiating paroxysmal atrial fibrillation: implication for catheter ablation. *J Am College Cardiol.* 2005;46(6):1054-1059.

20. Lin W-S, Tai C-T, Hsieh M-H, et al. Catheter ablation of paroxysmal atrial fibrillation initiated by non-pulmonary vein ectopy. *Circulation.* 2003;107(25):3176-3183.

21. Oral H, Chugh A, Good E, et al. A tailored approach to catheter ablation of paroxysmal atrial fibrillation. *Circulation.* 2006;113(15):1824-1831.

22. Nitta T, Ishii Y, Miyagi Y. Concurrent multiple left atrial focal activations with fibrillatory conduction and right atrial focal or reentrant activation as the mechanism in atrial fibrillation. *J Thorac Cardiovasc Surg.* 2004;127:770-778.

23. Yamauchi S, Ogasawara H, Saji Y. Efficacy of intraoperative mapping to optimize the surgical ablation of atrial fibrillation in cardiac surgery. *Ann Thorac Surg.* 2002;74: 450-457.

24. Harada A, Konishi T, Fukata M. Intraoperative map guided operation for atrial fibrillation due to mitral valve disease. *Ann Thorac Surg.* 2000;69:446-450.

25. Harada A, Sasake K, Fukushima T, et al. Atrial activation during chronic atrial fibrillation in patients with isolated mitral valve disease. *Ann Thorac Surg.* 1996;61:104-112.

26. Sueda T, Imai K, Ishii O. Efficacy of pulmonary vein isolation for the elimination of chronic atrial fibrillation in cardiac valvular surgery. *Ann Thorac Surg.* 2001;71: 1189-1193.

27. Schuessler RB. Do we need a map to get through the maze? *J Thorac Cardiovasc Surg.* 2004;127:627-628.

28. Kondo N, Takahashi K, Minakawa M. Left atrial maze procedure: a useful addition to other corrective operations. *Ann Thorac Surg.* 2003;75:1490-1494.

29. Gaita F, Gallotti R, Calo L. Limited posterior left atrial cryoablation in patients with chronic atrial fibrillation undergoing valvular heart sugery. *J Am Coll Cardiol.* 2000;36:159-166.

30. Tuinenburg AE, van Gelder IC, Tieleman R. Mini-maze suffices as adjunct to mitral valve surgery in patients with preoperative atrial fibrillation. *J Cardiovasc Electrophysiol.* 2000;11:960-967.

31. Kalil RAK, Lima GG, Leiria TLL, et al. Simple surgical isolation of pulmonary veins for treating secondary atrial fibrillation in mitral valve disease. *Ann Thorac Surg.* 2002;73(4): 1169-1173.

32. Deneke T, Khargi K, Grewe PH, et al. Left atrial versus bi-atrial Maze operation using intraoperatively cooled-tip radiofrequency ablation in patients undergoing open-heart surgery: safety and efficacy. *J Am College Cardiol.* 2002; 39(10):1644-1650.

33. Barnett SD, Ad N. Surgical ablation as treatment for the elimination of atrial fibrillation: a meta-analysis. *J Thorac Cardiovasc Surg.* 2006;131(5):1029-1035.

34. Calo L, Lamberti F, Loricchio ML, et al. Left atrial ablation versus biatrial ablation for persistent and permanent atrial fibrillation: a prospective and randomized study. *J Am College Cardiol.* 2006;47(12):2504-2512.

35. Usui A, Inden Y, Mizutani S. Repetitive atrial flutter as a complication of the left-sided simple maze procedure. *Ann Thorac Surg.* 2002;73:1457-1459.

36. Cox JL, Schuessler RB, Boineau JP. The development of the Maze procedure for the treatment of atrial fibrillation. *Semin Thorac Cardiovasc Surg.* 2000;12(1):2-14.

37. McCarthy PM, Gillinov AM, Castle L, Chung MK, Cosgrove Dr. The Cox–Maze procedure: the Cleveland clinic experience. *Semin Thorac Cardiovasc Surg.* 2000;12(1):25-29.

38. Schaff HV, Dearani JA, Daly RC, Orszulak TA, Danielson GK. Cox–Maze procedure for atrial fibrillation: Mayo clinic experience. *Semin Thorac Cardiovasc Surg.* 2000;12(1):30-37.

39. Prasad SM, Maniar HS, Camillo CJ, et al. The Cox maze III procedure for atrial fibrillation: long-term efficacy in patients undergoing lone versus concomitant procedures. *J Thorac Cardiovasc Surg.* 2003;126(6):1822-1828.

40. Cox JL, Ad N, Palazzo T. Impact of the maze procedure on the stroke rate in patients with atrial fibrillation. *J Thorac Cardiovasc Surg.* 1999;118:833-840.

41. Gillinov AM. Ablation of atrial fibrillation in mitral valve surgery. *Curr Opin Cardiol.* 2005;20:107-114.

42. Gillinov AM, Sirak JH, Blackstone EH. The Cox maze procedure in mitral valve disease: predictors of recurrent atrial fibrillation. *J Thorac Cardiovasc Surg.* 2005;130: 1653-1660.

43. Nitta T. Surgery for atrial fibrillation: a worldwide review. *Semin Thorac Cardiovasc Surg.* 2007;19(1):3-8.

44. Gaynor SL, Schuessler RB, Bailey MS, et al. Surgical treatment of atrial fibrillation: Predictors of late recurrence. *J Thorac Cardiovasc Surg.* 2005;129(1):104-111.

45. Scherer M, Dzemali O, Aybek T. Impact of left atrial size reduction on chronic atrial fibrillation in mitral valve surgery. *J Heart Valve Dis.* 2003;12:469-474.

46. Isobe F, Kawashima Y. The outcome and indications of the Cox maze III procedure for chronic atrial fibrillation with mitral valve disease. *J Thorac Cardiovasc Surg.* 1998; 116: 220-227.

47. Kawaguchi AT, Kosakai Y, Isobe F. Factors affecting rhythm after the Maze procedure for atrial fibrillation. *Circulation.* 1996;94:II-139-II-142.

48. Lee JW, Park NH, Choo SJ. Surgical outcome of the maze procedure for atrial fibrillation in mitral valve disease: rheumatic versus degenerative. *Ann Thorac Surg.* 2003; 75:57-61.

49. Jatene MB, Marcial MB, Tarasoutchi F. Influence of the maze procedure on the treatment of rheumatic atrial fibrillation – evaluation of rhythm control and clinical outcome in a comparative study. *Eur J Cardiothorac Surg.* 2000; 17:117-124.

50. Baek M-J, Na C-Y, Oh S-S, et al. Surgical treatment of chronic atrial fibrillation combined with rheumatic mitral valve disease: effects of the cryo-maze procedure and predictors for late recurrence. *Eur J Cardio-Thorac Surg.* 2006; 30(5):728-736.

51. Gillinov AM, Blackstone EH, McCarthy PM. Atrial fibrillation: current surgical options and their assessment. *Ann Thorac Surg.* 2002;74(6):2210-2217.

52. Gillinov AM, McCarthy PM. Advances in the surgical treatment of atrial fibrillation. *Cardiol Clin.* 2004;147-157.

53. Gillinov AM, McCarthy PM, Marrouche N, Natale A. Contemporary surgical treatment for atrial fibrillation. *Pacing Clin Electrophysiol.* 2003;26(7 Pt 2):1641-1644.

54. Raman J, Ishikawa S, Storer MM. Surgical radiofrequency ablation of both atria for atrial fibrillation: results of a multicenter trial. *J Thorac Cardiovasc Surg.* 2003;126: 1357-1366.

55. Sie HT, Beukema WP, Elvan A. Long-term results of irrigated radiofrequency modified maze procedure in 200 patients with concomitant cardiac surgery: six years experience. *Ann Thorac Surg.* 2004;77:512-516.

56. Luria DM, Nemec J, Etheridge SP. Intra-atrial conduction block along the mitral valve annulus during accessory pathway ablation: evidence for a left atrial "isthmus". *J Cardiovasc Electrophysiol.* 2001;12:744-749.

57. Cox JL, Ad N. The importance of cryoablation of the coronary sinus during the Maze procedure. *Semin Thorac Cardiovasc Surg.* 2000;12:20-24.

58. Gillinov AM, Saltman AE. Ablation of atrial fibrillation with concomitant cardiac surgery. *Semin Thorac Cardiovasc Surg.* 2007;19(1):25-32.

59. Nath S, Lynch Cd, Whayne JG, Haines DE. Cellular electrophysiological effects of hyperthermia on isolated guinea pig papillary muscle. Implications for catheter ablation. *Circulation.* 1993;88(4):1826-1831.

60. Lustgarten DL, Keane D, Ruskin J. Cryothermal ablation: mechanism of tissue injury and current experience in the treatment of tachyarrhythmias. *Prog Cardiovasc Dis.* 1999; 41(6):481-498.

61. Khargi K, Hutten BA, Lemke B, Deneke T. Surgical treatment of atrial fibrillation; a systematic review. *Eur J Cardiothorac Surg.* 2005;27(2):258-265.

62. Gillinov AM, Pettersson G, Rice TW. Esophageal injury during radiofrequency ablation for atrial fibrillation. *J Thorac Cardiovasc Surg.* 2001;122(6):1239-1240.

63. Doll N, Borger MA, Fabricius A, et al. Esophageal perforation during left atrial radiofrequency ablation: is the risk too high? *J Thorac Cardiovasc Surg.* 2003;125(4):836-842.

64. Manasse E, Medici D, Ghiselli S, Ornaghi D, Gallotti R. Left main coronary arterial lesion after microwave epicardial ablation. *Ann Thorac Surg.* 2003;76(1):276-277.

65. Johnson WD, Ganjoo AK, Stone CD. The left atrial appendage: our most lethal human attachment! Surgical implications. *Eur J Cardiothorac Surg.* 2000;17:718-722.

66. Garcia-Fernandez MA, Perez-David E, Quiles J. Role of left atrial appendage obliteration in stroke reduction in patients with mitral valve prosthesis: a transesophageal echocardiographic study. *J Am Coll Cardiol.* 2003;42: 1253-1258.

67. Rosenzweig BP, Katz E, Kort S. Thromboembolus from a ligated left atrial appendage. *J Am Soc Echocardiogr.* 2001; 14:396-398.

68. Gillinov AM, Pettersson BG, Dr C. Stapled excision of the left atrial appendage. *J Thorac Cardiovasc Surg.* 2004; 129: 679-680.

69. Pacifico A, Henry PD. Ablation for atrial fibrillation: are cures really achieved? *J Am Coll Cardiol.* 2004; 43: 1940-1942.

70. Saltman AE, Virmani R, Mohan A. Development and testing of a novel device for left atrial appendage occlusion. *Heart Surg Forum.* 2008;34:766-770.

71. Shemin RJ, Cox JL, Gillinov AM, Blackstone EH, Bridges CR. Guidelines for reporting data and outcomes for the surgical treatment of atrial fibrillation. *Ann Thorac Surg.* 2007; 83(3):1225-1230.

72. Doll N, Kiaii BB, Fabricius AM, et al. Intraoperative left atrial ablation (for atrial fibrillation) using a new argon cryocatheter: early clinical experience*1. *Ann Thorac Surg.* 2003;76(5 Suppl):1711-1715.

73. Mohr FW, Fabricius AM, Falk V, et al. Curative treatment of atrial fibrillation with intraoperative radiofrequency ablation: Short-term and midterm results. *J Thorac Cardiovasc Surg.* 2002;123(5):919-927.

74. Reade CC, Johnson JO, Bolotin G, et al. Combining robotic mitral valve repair and microwave atrial fibrillation ablation: techniques and initial results. *Ann Thorac Surg.* 2005; 79(2):480-484.

Gilles D. Dreyfus and Shahzad G. Raja

Tricuspid regurgitation (TR), until quite recently, has been considered and addressed only when severe; otherwise, it is barely referred to or totally ignored. TR can either be organic or functional (Table 15.1). In between, there are various combinations of these two well-defined pathologies.

Organic TR is defined as tricuspid valve incompetence with obvious structural abnormality of the tricuspid valve. This is best exemplified by rheumatic or carcinoid involvement of the tricuspid valve. Organic TR will not be discussed any further as valve replacement is more often indicated than repair, especially if symptoms are present along with moderate to severe TR.

Functional TR, on the other hand, is a term used to describe tricuspid valve incompetence without evident structural abnormality of the tricuspid valve. It is most commonly seen secondary to chronic mitral valve pathology, predominantly mitral regurgitation and frequently mitral stenosis.[1] It is also seen with aortic stenosis and often undermined or ignored.

Functional TR remains a debatable issue even in the current era. It seems that there is a consensus to treat severe TR when present along with left-sided lesions.[2] However, there is a marked variation in the treatment strategies for this entity and short- and long-term results are not comparable for these various techniques.

Natural History

The natural history of functional TR is quite clear; the increased left ventricular (LV) filling pressures progressively create an increase in pulmonary artery pressures, which in turn increase the right ventricular (RV) afterload.

The RV changes induce an annular dilatation, which in turn and with time will create a lack of leaflet coaptation and further, a leaflet tethering. Described as such, the underlying features that promote TR are easy to understand. However, RV changes are very complex and not similar to those seen in the LV.

The RV cannot sustain rapid changes in preload, afterload, or function. This setting is most obvious in RV infarction, which is not well tolerated clinically and hemodynamically and as such is often lethal.[3]

Conversely, the chronic RV changes are very well tolerated for a long time and even more surprising, some massive RV dilatation with a two or threefold increase in its size can still co-exist with a normal RV function. This setting is at best represented in Eisenmenger's syndrome, where pulmonary artery pressures can reach suprasystemic levels and yet will not provide TR.

Functional TR is regarded as a similar disease to functional mitral regurgitation (MR)[4] except for a long time and still until now spontaneous regression was believed to be a common pattern after surgical correction of left-sided disease. It is well accepted today that this concept is not true and that even functional TR can worsen on its own without identifiable contributing factors. Functional valve regurgitation could also be named as ventricular disease as it does not occur without structural and functional changes of the involved ventricle. However, once the LV function is impaired

G.D. Dreyfus (✉)
Medical Director of Cardio Thoracic Centre of Monaco,
11 bis, Avenue d'Ostende 98000, MONACO
e-mail: gdreyfus@ccm.mc

R.S. Bonser et al. (eds.), *Mitral Valve Surgery*,
DOI: 10.1007/978-1-84996-426-5_15, © Springer-Verlag London Limited 2011

Table 15.1 Causes of tricuspid regurgitation

Organic tricuspid regurgitation
- Rheumatic heart disease
- Endocarditis
- Ebstein anomaly
- Carcinoid
- Trauma
- Prolapse/myxomatous degeneration
- Segmental right ventricular disease (secondary to myocardial infarction, fibrosis, or infiltrative processes)
- Connective tissue diseases (Marfan syndrome, osteogenesis imperfecta, Ehlers-Danlos syndrome)
- Medications (methysergide, pergolide, fenfluramine)

Functional (secondary) tricuspid regurgitation
- Dilated cardiomyopathy of the right ventricle
- Left-sided valvular disease

and has resulted in functional MR, at a given time there will be no changes or minimal changes in LV shape, geometry, and function related to changes in preload and afterload. Conversely, once the RV has dilated or shown an impaired function, functional TR may increase or disappear in a very short time frame accordingly to major changes in shape, geometry, and function of the RV highly correlated to changes in preload and afterload.

Clinical Features

As functional TR is always, if not very often, related to left-sided lesions, these LV diseases provide symptoms that are predominant.

Except in extremely evolved RV dysfunction and/or severe TR, symptoms of TR are masked by those of the left-sided lesions. However, isolated severe TR can provide breathlessness and fatigue a bit like severe MR. We are more familiar with indirect signs of RV failure such as ascites, peripheral edema, and congestive hepatomegaly. At an advanced stage, liver and renal impairment become predominant with jaundice and elevated levels of biological markers of both these organs suggestive of end-stage disease that in itself becomes a contraindication to surgical intervention.

It is also to be stressed that for the management of symptoms of LV dysfunction, there are several pharmacological agents such as ACE inhibitors, beta blocking agents, calcium channel blockers, and

phosphodiesterase inhibitors. On the contrary, the pharmacological agents that are effective for relief of right heart failure symptoms are very limited, namely nitrates and diuretics. These facts have to be kept in mind when dealing with TR and/or RV dysfunction, as options for medical management are limited.

TR Assessment

TR assessment has remained quite superficial until recently, and in most echocardiography reports, it is just mentioned TR or no TR and the grading remains an eyeball judgment. Most reports do not mention anything about the structure and morphology of the leaflets, the annular size, and even less the RV size and function.

It seems quite important to bear in mind that TR grading is quite difficult and unreliable due to significant temporal variations in preload, afterload, RV size, and function. Hence, TR grading can change from one day to another, as these parameters may change altogether or independently one from the others!

As functional TR is a "ventricular disease" as well and not just a simple valvular disease,[4] there are two aspects of assessment of functional TR: assessment of tricuspid valve structure and function and assessment of right ventricular structure and function. Furthermore, accurate assessment of *functional tricuspid pathological process* must take into account the fact that there are three progressive stages. First or early stage is characterized by *annular dilatation with or without regurgitation;* second stage has *noncoapting leaflets* creating various degrees of regurgitation, with probably a greater degree of annular dilatation; and third stage is recognized by *leaflet tethering* which is a well-defined entity with a tenting height of at least 8 mm below the plane of the annulus.[4]

It is interesting to point out that assessment of functional TR has been a relatively ignored aspect at most centers worldwide. A simple parameter such as tricuspid annulus diameter (TAD) that has an important role in the TV surgical decision-making process is rarely measured preoperatively as a routine. Using two-dimensional echocardiography, TAD is obtained from the apical four-chamber (AP4CH) and parasternal short axis (PSAX) views at an end-diastolic and end-systolic still frame (Fig. 15.1a). It is defined as the distance between the insertion sites of septal and anterior TV leaflets.[5] There is a trend to believe that the tricuspid annulus is dilated if the TAD is >40 mm or 21 mm/m[2,6,7] However, it is important to emphasize that there is a significant discrepancy between preoperative and intraoperative measurement of TAD[8] (Fig. 15.1).

Coaptation height is the other important parameter that must be taken into account when assessing tricuspid valve morphology. Coaptation takes place at the level of the plane of the annulus. If coaptation height is <2 mm or an edge-to-edge coaptation is used, then the likelihood of developing further regurgitation is very high.[8] This is reflective of lesser degree of RV dilatation. In this setting, the presence or the absence of regurgitation should not lead to the conclusion that there is no tricuspid disease.

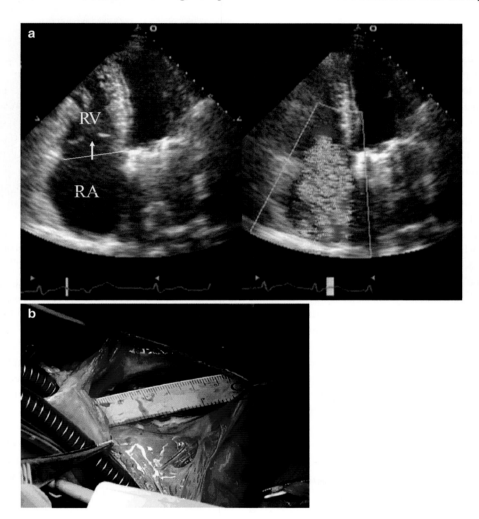

Fig. 15.1 (**a**) The modified apical 4 chambers view (when the P3 and A3 are seen at level of mitral valve) is the most accurate view to asses the dimension of tricuspid annulus but even like this the discrepancy is frequently observed. Anwar et al.[14] demonstrated that the tricuspid annulus shape is not circular but oval and it has a minor and a major diameter and In fact in AP4CH the measurement involve the minor not a major diameter of the annulus. The single echocardiographic view reliable to measure the major diameter is the transgastric view with right rotation by TEE. (**b**) Tricuspid annular plane systolic excursion (TAPSE) is the most frequently used index for evaluating RV function and it measures the extent of systolic motion of the tricuspid annullus towards the apex. Normale value in the literature is more than 14 mm. In the last period tissue Doppler imaging is a more and more frequently used technique to predict global right ventricle dysfunction. A value less than 11.5 cm/ s for tricuspid annulus velocities is able to predict a global dysfonction of right ventricle with EF RV <45 %.[35] The main disadvantage of this modality is necesity to have a good alignment with the ultrasound beam. Another parameter derived from Doppler myocardial imaging is myocardial isovolumic acceleration time (IVA) a parameter less dependent ofloading. An IVA value at level of basal segment of RV free wall of >1.1 m/s[2] correlates with MRI RVEF >45%[36]

These are the patients who with minor alterations in hemodynamics of the RV will manifest significant TR.

Second subset of patients as previously mentioned have annular dilatation, central lack of coaptation, with some degree of restricted leaflet motion, and virtual coaptation taking place at the level of the annulus to within 8 mm of the plane of the annulus. This group of patients will have moderate to severe TR again influenced by the RV hemodynamics.

Third subset of patients have some degree of annular dilatation and greater degree of restricted leaflet motion that is enhanced by the tethering of the free edges of the leaflets, predominantly the anterior leaflet, due to the specific anatomical features of the RV. This subset is now acknowledged as a separate entity and is being assessed using sophisticated echocardiographic parameters including end-systolic RV eccentricity index, RV sphericity index, and tricuspid valve tethering area.[4,9]

RV long-axis length and RV short-axis width measured at the mid-ventricular level are used to calculate the RV sphericity index at end-systole and end-diastole(Fig. 15.2).[10] Tricuspid valve tethering area (Fig. 15.3) is measured by the area between the atrial surface of the leaflets and the annulus plane at end-systole.[11]

In fact, end-systolic RV eccentricity index, TV tethering area, and end-diastolic tricuspid annulus diameter are independently related to effective regurgitant orifice area (EROA) of the tricuspid valve in patients with chronic RV dilation, further strengthening the concept that functional TR is a ventricular disease and RV geometric change independently determines functional TR severity.[4]

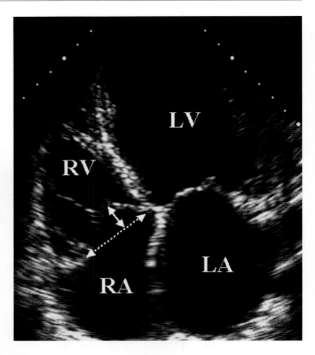

Fig. 15.3 Diagram of apical four-chamber view demonstrating technique of measurements of distance and area of tricuspid valve (TV) tethering. TV tethering distance is indicated by the distance between the tips of arrowheads (*solid line*). Segmentation schema of oblique line is used for measurement of area of TV tethering. The broken line with arrowheads is the tricuspid annulus diameter as measured on two-dimensional echocardiography. LA indicates left atrium

Two-dimensional (2D) echocardiography, M-mode and tissue Doppler recording are the commonly employed modalities for the assessment of tricuspid valve structure and function. Although two-dimensional echocardiography is helpful to assess TV function and to detect TR severity (Fig. 15.1b).[5,12]

Cardiovascular magnetic resonance imaging (CMRI) and real-time three-dimensional echocardiography (RT3DE) are currently emerging as more accurate and informative diagnostic modalities for evaluating the TV more completely.[5,13] Both CMRI and RT3DE may yield more detailed anatomical description of TA morphology and function.[13,14] Furthermore, accurate assessment of RV, especially in the setting of RV dilatation or in cases of depressed RV function, is difficult with routine two-dimensional echocardiography. Therefore, CMRI has a definite role in the detailed assessment of RV function, with special emphasis on calculation of regurgitant volume, stroke volume, end-systolic volume, end-diastolic volume,

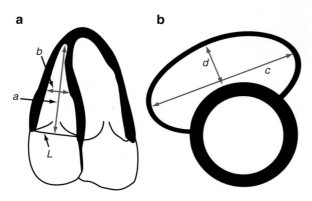

Fig. 15.2 Difference in measurement of tricuspid annular diameter. (**a**) Preoperatively > 4 cm. (**b**) Intraoperatively > 7 cm

and ejection fraction. In our personal experience, we have found by CMRI that some right ventricles with a three- to fourfold volume increase above normal were still able to maintain normal ejection fraction, which emphasizes how different are LV and RV changes and their meanings.

Surgical Treatment

Surgical treatment of functional TR is still not standardized and is under debate; this remains true for the type of surgical procedure as for the type of annuloplasty and finally is reflected by heterogeneous surgical results (Tables 15.2 and 15.3).

Surgery can either be a valve replacement or a tricuspid repair, which until recently was limited to a simple annuloplasty.

Valve replacement should have no room in functional TR except in cases of severely dilated RV along with tethered leaflets. If that should be the case, bioprosthetic replacement is far safer than mechanical replacement provided that low gradients across the tricuspid orifice are ensured by implanting the biggest valve possible (size 31–33 mm), irrespective of the body surface area of the patient.

Valve repair is by far the preferable option, which provides quite good results. To undertake successful valve repair, consideration is given to two parameters: annular dilatation and presence or absence of tethering.

Annuloplasty addresses annular dilatation and can be achieved by different means.

De Vega technique is the traditional annuloplasty that consists of plication of the posterior and anterior portion of the annulus, preserving the septal portion, with a double continuous suture.[15] This was the first systematic approach to treat TR by reducing the size of the tricuspid annulus and has provided fairly good early results[16–20] and more questionable long-term results.[21] It is quick to perform and inexpensive. It was designed to treat moderate annular dilatation as stated by De Vega himself. It is not, however, indicated for severe annular dilatation. Two inherent complications of this technique need highlighting. An early complication is undersizing of the tricuspid orifice, thereby creating tricuspid stenosis, which is extremely difficult to recognize, and a later complication is fibrotic retraction of the leaflets on the running suture called the guitar-string effect that leads to recurrent regurgitation and exposes the patient to subsequent tricuspid replacement as re-repair is no longer feasible.

Two other techniques that have been reported to be effective for treating functional TR include the clover technique[22] and the modified suture bicuspidization technique.[23] De Bonis et al.[22] reported the clover technique, which consists of stitching together the central part of the free edges of the leaflets producing a "clover"-shaped valve. A modified version of suture bicuspidization, originally described by Kay, Maselli-Campagna, and Tsuji in 1965,[24] as a technique to correct TR has also been reported by Ghanta et al. to be

Table 15.2 Current outcomes of tricuspid valve replacement

Author, Year	Type of prosthetic valve		Follow-up years	Actuarial survival %	Freedom from valve-related events %	Freedom from structural valve deterioration %	Freedom from reoperation %
	Biological	Mechanical					
Tokunaga et al., 2008	27	4	15	75.6	84.9	85.7	NA
Chang et al., 2006	35	103	15	73.8 ± 8.5	49.9 ± 8.0	NA	66.3 ± 9.4
Filsoufi et al., 2005	34	47	5	45[a], 59[b]	100[a], 80[b]	80[a,b]	100[a], 98[b]
Carrier et al., 2003	82	15	4 ± 5	56 ± 6[a], 60 ± 13[b]	94[b]	92[a]	91 ± 9[a], 91 ± 9[b]
Kaplan et al., 2002	32	97	20	65.1 ± 9.3	92.6 ± 6.9	90 ± 5.5[a], 97.8 ± 4.2[b]	NA

NA = not available; [a] = Bioprosthesis; [b] = Mechanical prosthesis

Table 15.3 Current outcomes of tricuspid valve repair

Author, Year	Technique(s)	Number of patients	Follow-up years %	Survival %	In-hospital mortality %	Prevalence of grade 3+/4%+ TR %	Reoperation rate %
Ghanta et al., 2007	Suture bicuspidization	157	3	75.3	6.4	6/8	1.9
	Ring annuloplasty	80		61.2	11.3	7/10	
Gatti et al., 2007	Koehler band	53	19.2 ±1 4.0 months	91.7	5.7	0	0
Filsoufi et al., 2006	Edwards MC3 system	51	6 months	82.5	3.8	NA	0
Dreyfus et al., 2005	Carpentier-Edwards classic ring	148	10	90.3	0.6	0.7	0
McCarthy et al., 2004	Carpentier-Edwards semirigid ring	139	8	50	8	11	3
	Cosgrove-Edwards flexible band	291				6	
	De Vega procedure	116				20	
	Peri-Guard	243				22	
Carrier et al., 2004	De Vega procedure	107	15	30 ± 6	NA	NA	37 ± 2[a]
	Bex linear reducer	256	15	35 ± 5			33 ± 1
	Carpentier-Edwards semirigid ring	89	5	88 ± 4			5 ± 7
De Bonis et al., 2003	Clover technique	14	2	92.9	7.1	0	0
Onoda et al., 2000	Carpentier-Edwards semirigid ring	45	10	68.3	6.6	NA	2.5

[a]Median freedom rate from tricuspid repair failure (clinical right heart failure, redo annuloplasty, tricuspid valve replacement at follow-up)
NA = not available

an effective, inexpensive, and simple-to-perform strategy for tackling moderate functional TR.[23] This relatively simple technique involves figure-of-eight suture plication of the posterior leaflet to reduce annulus size.

The other more reliable option for treatment of functional TR is the use of prosthetic ring annuloplasty. The concept of ring annuloplasty was developed by Carpentier and is based on reshaping concept rather than shrinking the tricuspid annulus.[25] Choosing the appropriate-sized ring depends on the measurement of the unfolded anterior leaflet. The ring is secured by mattress 3/0 nonabsorbable, braided suture. The oval tricuspid annuloplasty ring is semiflexible, conforms to the configuration of the normal tricuspid orifice, and has an opening in the anteroseptal commissure that

allows surgeons to avoid sutures in the area of the Bundle of His. Hence, there is no increased incidence of conduction disturbances.

A modified version especially designed for the American market is the MC[3] annuloplasty ring. It has a three-dimensional design, is rigid, and is preconfigured to accommodate the saddle shape of the annulus.[26]

Other prosthetic substitutes such as customized semicircular Peri-Guard annuloplasty,[21] Cosgrove band[21,27] and Koehler band[28] have also been used. Recently, McCarthy and colleagues reported the Cleveland Clinic experience including 790 patients who underwent a tricuspid valve annuloplasty using four different techniques (i.e., the De Vega repair, the pericardial patch, the Cosgrove flexible band [Edwards LifeSciences], and the Carpentier-Edwards ring [Edwards LifeSciences]).[21] Similar to the previous studies,[29,30] this clinical series also confirmed the superiority of prosthetic annuloplasty over other repair techniques. However, an important finding of McCarthy and colleagues'[21] study was the fact that a tricuspid annuloplasty did not consistently eliminate functional TR. The authors reported the presence of significant residual TR (i.e., 3+ to 4+) at 1 month in about 15% of patients who underwent a prosthetic annuloplasty.

The study by McCarthy et al.[21] highlights the concept that we have routinely practiced for the treatment of functional TR. This concept emphasizes that different surgical techniques are required for effective treatment of functional TR for the three subsets of patients as previously described in this manuscript. Our approach is outlined below.

Patients with Annular Dilatation with or Without Regurgitation

This is the only subset in which any annuloplasty technique will provide excellent results. However, we favor the use of an annuloplasty ring because the use of a prosthetic ring allows a tailored reshaping of the annulus and most likely will provide best long-term results. This view of ours is supported by our publication,[8] in which we have dealt with the problem of secondary tricuspid dilatation, with or without regurgitation. We have reported outcomes for 311 patients who underwent mitral valve repair (MVR). The tricuspid valve was examined in each patient. Tricuspid annuloplasty was performed only if the tricuspid annular diameter was greater than twice the normal size ($\geq$70 mm) regardless of the grade of regurgitation. Patients in group 1 (163 patients; 52.4%) received MVR alone. Patients in group 2 (148 patients; 47.6%) received MVR plus tricuspid annuloplasty. Although not significant, there was a difference with regard to hospital mortality (group 1 = 1.8%, group 2 = 0.7%) and actuarial survival rate (Kaplan–Meier: group 1 = 97.3%, 96.2%, and 85.5%; group 2 = 98.5%, 98.5%, and 90.3% at 3, 5, and 10 years, respectively). The New York Heart Association (NYHA) functional class was significantly improved in group 2 (group 1 = 1.59 ± 0.84; group 2 = 1.11 ± 0.31; $p1$). TR increased by more than two grades in 48% of the patients in group 1 (patients

without annuloplasty) and in only 2% of the patients in group 2 ($p < 0.001$). Actuarial long-term survival was better in patients who received an annuloplasty ring, although did not reach statistical significance. We have, based on the findings of this study, concluded that remodeling annuloplasty of the tricuspid valve based on tricuspid dilation improves functional status irrespective of the grade of regurgitation. Considerable tricuspid dilatation can be present even in the absence of substantial TR. Tricuspid dilatation is an ongoing disease process that will, with time, lead to severe TR. In other words, we are proposing "prophylactic" annuloplasty in order to avoid progression of the disease. It does also avoid the unsolvable dilemma of isolated severe residual TR, which still carries out an operative mortality of 30–50% and has no agreed guidelines for indication and timing for surgery. This concept has been acknowledged and incorporated into the recent guidelines from the American College of Cardiology (ACC) and American Heart Association (AHA).[31]

Patients with Annular Dilatation with Moderate or Severe TR with Some Degree of Tethering

This subset is always treated with ring annuloplasty and probably an undersized ring by one or two sizes in order to overcome the tethering component.

Patients with Annular Dilatation with Severe Tethering

In this subgroup, tethering becomes the major component. Interestingly, this entity had not been recognized until recently and therefore had not been addressed in a specific manner. For these patients, until recently only two options were available: (a) standard undersized annuloplasty and (b) tricuspid valve replacement.

Standard undersized annuloplasty is associated with a significant incidence of residual/recurrent TR in this subset of patients.[21,32,33] We have developed a new technique for this entity.[34] This innovative and easily reproducible technique uses autologous pericardial patch to extend the anterior leaflet of tricuspid valve.

The rationale for this technique is that in the presence of significant tethering, especially in the context of RV dilatation, which is quite different from that of the LV, the changes of shape and the extent of tethering are not really predictable. There are two surgical options: an undersized annuloplasty, which aims to try to overcome the tethering by achieving a forced coaptation at the level of the annulus. We already know that this theory has its limitations on the left side of the heart despite the predictable size of a loaded left ventricle and virtually no changes in its size according to various conditions. Hence, in the case of unpredictable RV geometric changes, it will not be an effective option. The other option is to bring the coaptation down deep into the ventricle due to the tethering. Looking at the echocardiograms of such patients, the lack of tissue of the leaflets is obvious, in relation to a massive annular dilatation and tethering >8 mm. By combining both the reduction in annular size and a dramatic increase in the leaflet size, we have been able to treat successfully this entity of significant leaflet tethering in a significant number of patients.

Conclusion

The right ventricle is a complex entity that has been undermined for a long time. There is a growing interest in the recent era in the right ventricle along with its most easily accessible marker, the tricuspid valve and its regurgitation. Indications for surgery for tricuspid disease, annulus or leaflet, has yet not reached a consensus. However, there is an overall agreement that it has been undertreated and that more careful analysis should be carried out for effective surgical management of this condition, which is accountable for a higher morbidity and mortality than is generally expected.

References

1. Hannoush H, Fawzy ME, Stefadouros M, et al. Regression of significant tricuspid regurgitation after mitral balloon valvotomy for severe mitral stenosis. *Am Heart J.* 2004; 148:865-870.
2. Kuwaki K, Morishita K, Tsukamoto M, et al. Tricuspid valve surgery for functional tricuspid valve regurgitation associated with left-sided valvular disease. *Eur J Cardiothorac Surg.* 2001;20:577-582.
3. Pfisterer M. Right ventricular involvement in myocardial infarction and cardiogenic shock. *Lancet.* 2003;362:392-394.
4. Kim HK, Kim YJ, Park JS, et al. Determinants of the severity of functional tricuspid regurgitation. *Am J Cardiol.* 2006; 98:236-242.
5. Anwar AM, Soliman OI, Nemes A, et al. Value of assessment of tricuspid annulus: real-time three-dimensional echocardiography and magnetic resonance imaging. *Int J Cardiovasc Imaging.* 2007;23:701-705.
6. Colombo T, Russo C, Ciliberto GR, et al. Tricuspid regurgitation secondary to mitral valve disease: tricuspid annulus function as guide to tricuspid valve repair. *Cardiovasc Surg.* 2001;9:369-377.
7. Antunes MJ, Barlow JB. Management of tricuspid valve regurgitation. *Heart.* 2007;93:271-276.
8. Dreyfus GD, Corbi PJ, Chan KM, et al. Secondary tricuspid regurgitation or dilatation: which should be the criteria for surgical repair? *Ann Thorac Surg.* 2005;79:127-132.
9. Fukuda S, Gillinov AM, Song JM, et al. Echocardiographic insights into atrial and ventricular mechanisms of functional tricuspid regurgitation. *Am Heart J.* 2006;152:1208-1214.
10. Reynertson SI, Kundur R, Mullen GM, et al. Asymmetry of right ventricular enlargement in response to tricuspid regurgitation. *Circulation.* 1999;100:465-467.
11. Sagie A, Schwammenthal E, Padial LR, et al. Determinants of functional tricuspid regurgitation in incomplete tricuspid valve closure: Doppler color flow study of 109 patients. *J Am Coll Cardiol.* 1994;24:446-453.
12. Schnabel R, Khaw AV, von Bardeleben RS, et al. Assessment of the tricuspid valve morphology by transthoracic real-time-3D-echocardiography. *Echocardiography.* 2005;22: 15-23.
13. Fukuda S, Saracino G, Matsumura Y, et al. Three-dimensional geometry of the tricuspid annulus in healthy subjects and in patients with functional tricuspid regurgitation: a real-time, 3-dimensional echocardiographic study. *Circulation.* 2006; 114(1 Suppl):I492-I498.
14. Anwar AM, Geleijnse ML, Ten Cate FJ, Meijboom FJ. Assessment of tricuspid valve annulus size, shape and function using real-time three-dimensional echocardiography. *Interact Cardiovasc Thorac Surg* 2006;5:683-7.
15. De Vega NG. Selective, adjustable and permanent annuloplasty. An original technic for the treatment of tricuspid insufficiency. *Rev Esp Cardiol.* 1972;25:555-556. Spanish.
16. Rabago G, De Vega NG, Castillon L, et al. The new De Vega technique in tricuspid annuloplasty (results in 150 patients). *J Cardiovasc Surg (Torino).* 1980;21:231-238.
17. Iwa T, Watanabe Y, Tsuchiya K, et al. Improved surgical treatment of tricuspid insufficiency in combined valvular diseases. *J Cardiovasc Surg (Torino).* 1980;21:604-613.
18. Holper K, Haehnel JC, Augustin N, et al. Surgery for tricuspid insufficiency: long-term follow-up after De Vega annuloplasty. *Thorac Cardiovasc Surg.* 1993;41:1-8.
19. Carrier M, Pellerin M, Guertin MC, et al. Twenty-five years' clinical experience with repair of tricuspid insufficiency. *J Heart Valve Dis.* 2004;13:952-956.
20. De Paulis R, Bobbio M, Ottino G, et al. The De Vega tricuspid annuloplasty. Perioperative mortality and long-term follow-up. *J Cardiovasc Surg (Torino).* 1990;31:512-517.
21. McCarthy PM, Bhudia SK, Rajeswaran J, et al. Tricuspid valve repair: durability and risk factors for failure. *J Thorac Cardiovasc Surg.* 2004;127:674-685.

22. De Bonis M, Lapenna E, La Canna G, et al. A novel technique for correction of severe tricuspid valve regurgitation due to complex lesions. *Eur J Cardiothorac Surg*. 2004;25: 760-765.

23. Ghanta RK, Chen R, Narayanasamy N, et al. Suture bicuspidization of the tricuspid valve versus ring annuloplasty for repair of functional tricuspid regurgitation: midterm results of 237 consecutive patients. *J Thorac Cardiovasc Surg*. 2007;133:117-126.

24. Kay JH, Maselli-Campagna G, Tsuji KK. Surgical treatment of tricuspid insufficiency. *Ann Surg*. 1965;162:53-58.

25. Deloche A, Guérinon J, Fabiani JN, et al. Anatomical study of rheumatic tricuspid valvulopathies. Applications to the critical study of various methods of annuloplasty. *Arch Mal Coeur Vaiss*. 1974;67:497-505. French.

26. Filsoufi F, Salzberg SP, Coutu M, et al. A three-dimensional ring annuloplasty for the treatment of tricuspid regurgitation. *Ann Thorac Surg*. 2006;81:2273-2277.

27. Gatti G, Maffei G, Lusa AM, et al. Tricuspid valve repair with the Cosgrove-Edwards annuloplasty system: early clinical and echocardiographic results. *Ann Thorac Surg*. 2001;72:764-767.

28. Gatti G, Marcianò F, Antonini-Canterin F, et al. Tricuspid valve annuloplasty with a flexible prosthetic band. *Interact Cardiovasc Thorac Surg*. 2007;6:731-735.

29. Rivera R, Duran E, Ajuria M. Carpentier's flexible ring versus De Vega's annuloplasty. A prospective randomized study. *J Thorac Cardiovasc Surg*. 1985;89:196-203.

30. Matsuyama K, Matsumoto M, Sugita T, et al. De Vega annuloplasty and Carpentier-Edwards ring annuloplasty for secondary tricuspid regurgitation. *J Heart Valve Dis*. 2001; 10:520-524.

31. American College of Cardiology/American Heart Association Task Force on Practice Guidelines; Society of Cardiovascular Anesthesiologists; Society for Cardiovascular Angiography and Interventions; Society of Thoracic Surgeons, Bonow RO, Carabello BA, Kanu C, et al. ACC/AHA 2006 guidelines for the management of patients with valvular heart disease: a report of the American College of Cardiology/American Heart Association Task Force on Practice Guidelines (writing committee to revise the 1998 Guidelines for the Management of Patients With Valvular Heart Disease): developed in collaboration with the Society of Cardiovascular Anesthesiologists: endorsed by the Society for Cardiovascular Angiography and Interventions and the Society of Thoracic Surgeons. *Circulation*. 2006;114:e84-e231.

32. Fukuda S, Gillinov AM, McCarthy PM, et al. Determinants of recurrent or residual functional tricuspid regurgitation after tricuspid annuloplasty. *Circulation*. 2006;114: I582-I587.

33. Matsunaga A, Duran CM. Progression of tricuspid regurgitation after repaired functional ischemic mitral regurgitation. *Circulation*. 2005;112(9 Suppl):I453-I457.

34. Dreyfus GD, Raja SG, Chan KMJ. Tricuspid leaflet extension to address severe tethering in functional tricuspid regurgitation. *Eur J Cardiothorac Surg*. 2008;34:908-910. doi: 10.1016/j.ejcts.2008.07.006 9.

35. Meluzin J, Spinarova L, Bakala J, Toman J, Krejci J, Hude P, et al. Pulsed Doppler tissue imaging of the velocity of tricuspid annular systolic motion. A new, rapid, and non-invasive method of evaluating right ventricular systolic function. *Eur Heart J* 2001;22:340-8.

36. Jenkins C, Chan J, Bricknell K, Strudwick M, Marwick TH. Reproducibility of right ventricular volumes and ejection fraction using real-time three-dimensional echocardiography: comparison with cardiac MRI. *Chest* 2007;131: 1844-51.

Index

R.S. Bonser et al. (eds.), *Mitral Valve Surgery*,
DOI: 10.1007/978-1-84996-426-5, © Springer-Verlag London Limited 2011